PREFACE

The need has been felt for some time for a current book on spectacle frames, and their general context within the field of ocular dispensing. Sasieni's classic book on *Spectacle Fitting and Optical Dispensing* was published in 1950. This was brought up to date and largely re-written under the title of *Principles and Practice of Optical Dispensing and Fitting* in 1962.

Optical students in particular have felt the need for such a book, but with the bewildering variety of frames which have become available, and the increasingly international nature of the design and distribution of frames, practising opticians are probably no less in need of advice where relevant.

The book has deliberately been kept as brief as possible, and in many respects it is too brief. I am aware of this, but the whole concept is to provide principle rather than practice, in a subject which is essentially practical in nature. The result is a compromise, often at times not a very satisfactory one. Further the application of principle to practice in 1970 will not be the same in a few years' time when a new generation of frame styles will have made their debut—and possibly exit also (for fashion is notoriously fickle).

I am indebted to my colleagues, Mr. R. W. Butler, and particularly Mr. E. Ford, for helpful suggestions and comments in the preparation of the text. Various other persons have been very helpful, and I should mention in particular Mr. B. Green of Birch-Stigmat Ltd., Mr. A. W. Tyler of Merx Optical Co. Ltd., and Mr. A. E. R. Buckle of Clement Clarke Ltd.

The following companies have kindly given me permission to use frames and illustrations as necessary:-
Oliver Goldsmith Ltd., M. Bender Ltd., British American Optical Co. Ltd., Martin Wells Pty., M. Wiseman Ltd., Highgate Optical Co. Ltd., Look Designs Ltd., Societe des Lunetiers, Anglo-American Optical Co. Ltd., Knight Optical Co. Ltd., Trident Optical Co. Ltd., Grafton Optical Co. Ltd., Connaught Investments, Societe Industrielle de Lunetterie.

The British Standards Institution have kindly given me permission to reproduce the sections of B.S. 3199 as an appendix to Ch. II.

Mr. M. G. Aird has been unceasing in his efforts to enable this book to be published, and I am grateful to him and to the Association of Dispensing Opticians for undertaking the publication.

Finally my thanks are due to the various persons who acted as models for the photographs in illustration of the various aspects of this work. Without their active cooperation, I could not have accomplished what was required.

London, 1970   G. H. CLAYTON.

GW01465144

i

CONTENTS

v

CHAPTER I

SPECTACLE FRAMES AND MATERIALS

1.1. Introduction

1.1A. We are concerned in this book with the practical aspect of frames and their measurement. We are also concerned with the determination of certain facial measurements and in particular with the position of the eyes in the head. Technical matters concerned with ophthalmic lenses, the behaviour of light on passing through lenses, and so on, do not require our attention at this time, except in so far as the dispensing of the complete spectacles is concerned. In this context we are interested mainly in the positioning of the lenses in the frames.

Ophthalmic dispensing consists of supplying a frame that will enable the required pair of lenses to be fitted in a comfortable and optically satisfactory position in front of the eyes. The main emphasis when dispensing must be directed towards the lenses, but since the frames are the means by which the lenses are held in place to enable the patient to see, it is vitally important that each of these two aspects of our work, both frames and lenses, shall receive the necessary attention.

This book is directed mainly towards frame dispensing, and although certain aspects of lens dispensing are discussed, particularly the positioning of the lenses in the frame, or the positioning of the lenses before the eyes, this is not the main purpose.

The usual manner in which spectacle dispensing is undertaken is for the optician to order a frame from his supplier to be glazed with the necessary lenses. The supplier may be either (a) a Prescription House which will make or obtain the necessary frame from the actual manufacturer, and will then glaze it with the required lenses, or (b) the frame manufacturer who will send the empty frame which will then be subsequently glazed. It may be that a sample frame which the optician has already, perhaps in stock or for display purposes, may be satisfactory and can be used for the patient. This latter procedure has much to recommend it, for the person is able to see exactly what is being supplied, and furthermore the frame is immediately available.

1

1.1B. Frame fitting is essentially and mainly an art, and only secondarily a science. A frame *may* be fitted solely with reference to a set of facial measurements. In practice it seldom is. An optician requiring a frame for his client stipulates on his order firstly a style of frame and than a set of measurements required for that frame.

1.1C. Facial measurements may be made with rulers (also termed "rules") but these measurements must be modified as required to such different frames as may be selected. The same face may require somewhat different measurements for different frames to be fitted comfortably and accurately.

1.1D. In many countries of the world a set of standards is laid down. In Great Britain, these standards are listed as B.S.3199 (measurement of spectacles), which is reproduced in Ch. 2 for reference. Reference might also be made to B.S. 3521 (Glossary of Terms relating to Ophthalmic Lenses and Spectacles) which is an invaluable source of information upon the same topic.

1.1E. In spite of the detailed nature of these standards, it is found that the same measurement (ostensibly) will vary from one frame to the next to an alarming extent. This means that the optician must not only be aware of these standards, but also of the way in which they are applied in the various frames he supplies. Again this means that a set of measurements taken for a frame made by one manufacturer, will require modification if an apparently similar frame is made by another manufacturer.

1.1F. Many frames are only made in a limited range of sizes and colour.

1.1G. Since the sizes and their range vary from frame to frame and manufacturer to manufacturer, it is essential for the optician to become familiar with the products of each manufacturer. Perhaps since it is impossible to be conversant with the whole range of any one manufacturer, it might be advisable to say that it is essential to become familiar with the range and size of the particular frames that the optician normally handles. See Chapters 4 and 5.

1.1H. There are various objectives to be borne in mind when fitting spectacle frames. Which of these objectives will be paramount in any one case will depend on the merits of the particular case. The following points must be observed:

    (a) optical requirements for the lenses which are needed.
    (b) appearance.
    (c) comfort in wear.
    (d) special facial measurements.
    (e) rigidity and/or physical strength of frame
    (f) anticipated life of frame.

Undoubtedly there are many other objectives which the optician might have in mind from time to time depending upon the circumstances involved, but the above list enumerates the most important.

1.1J. In Great Britain and in other countries where similar schemes exist the National Health Service has a very inhibiting influence upon the frame styles and lenses available, and consequently upon the measurements required.

1.2. "Spectacle frames are expected to last forever"

This paragraph should be interpreted somewhat humorously, although as all opticians are aware from bitter experience, much friction is caused by the factors stated below. Unfortunately it appears to be tacitly assumed by most of the general public that a spectacle frame bears a generic resemblance to a set of dentures. It is supplied by someone who has some vague connection with the medical world. It is expected to last for ever, for all purposes—or at least until it wears out at some indeterminate date in the future. If broken, it is expected that facilities will be available for immediate repair.

It is our duty as opticians to educate the public to the advisibility of alternative spectacles for different purposes (other than distance and near when presbyopia has set in), and to give them to understand that with the best will in the world we are often quite unable to mend a broken frame immediately, or replace a broken lens at once. A spare pair therefore is an urgent physical necessity.

1.3. Materials used in Spectacle Manufacturing

There are various materials used for spectacle frames, the most important of which are as follows:-

(a) TORTOISESHELL, being the shell of the hawks-bill turtle. It comes mainly from the West Indies, is now rather rare, and consequently more costly. The advantages are lightness of weight, beautiful polish and finish that can be imparted to it, exclusiveness and rarity appeal, and occasionally as an alternative to a plastics material where there is a skin allergy. If broken, frames can sometimes be repaired by splicing.

(b) PLASTICS. *N.B.* The use of the word "plastics" and not "plastic" is deliberate in this context, as "plastic" as an adjective means in a semi-solid or semi-fluid state, or even pliable and flexible of a solid. When referring to spectacle frames, "plastics" will be used.

There are two main types, thermoplastic (or thermosoftening) and thermosetting (or thermohardening). Examples of the former are cellulose

3

acetate and cellulose nitrate. Acetate material is the most widely used in Gt. Britain as it discolours less than nitrate, is more easily worked, lenses may be "sprung-in" more easily, it takes dyes more readily, layers of material may be fused or stuck together more readily, and it lasts longer in wear. Nitrate is inflammable and discolours more readily, but is harder and less liable to warp in wear.

The acrylic resins (perspex) are thermosetting, and these are usually harder, more brilliantly coloured, will withstand higher temperatures, and are less liable to be affected by chemical action (notably body acids) than the cellulose range. They will however break more easily.

The above are brief details of the plastics materials used in frame manufacture. Below, these details have been elaborated somewhat to provide additional information.

Thermoplastic materials for spectacle frame manufacturing have been in use almost since the beginning of the plastics industry. For example "lactoid" which was made from milk, was in use in the early 1930s. Cellulose acetate and cellulose nitrate are probably the best known of such materials, and are produced synthetically from organic sources, usually wood pulp and cotton linters (fibres which are too short for spinning). These cellulose materials have a fairly low softening point of about 65°C.

Some little time before 1939 the plastics industry began a rapid expansion when it was found possible to produce the raw materials from coal and petroleum, as by-products. Several materials were produced, which have limited application for spectacle frames. Polystyrene is one, but this is not suitable because of certain physical properties, e.g. the surface is very soft and is attacked by petrol and acetone. The vinyls are another of the thermoplastics which can and have been used.

In Gt. Britain cellulose nitrate is not very much used for spectacle wear, although elsewhere its use is more widespread but still limited. Usually this is the state in tropical countries where its hardness and lesser tendency to warping is an advantage. However its tendency to discolouration and proneness to attack by body acids (a condition obviously exacerbated by heat and humidity) tend to reduce the advantages somewhat. Cellulose nitrate is more generally used when a certain amount of machining is required, e.g. hoods on a metal combination frame, because it is dimensionally more stable than acetate.

Cellulose acetate is available in two forms, known as sliced acetate and extruded acetate. New techniques and methods of production have produced a better product in the extruded form which is more suitable for spectacle frames.

In order to produce sliced acetate slabs for spectacle frame production, acetate granules softened with solvent and plasticiser are squeezed between rollers to form thin sheets of a given colour. These sheets which contain a high proportion of plasticiser and solvent are stacked with alternate colours depending on the final pattern required. Also depending on the final pattern, strips are used to build up a layer, rather than complete sheets.

The stack of sheets is then subjected to hydraulic pressure which together with the solvent and plasticiser action produce a homogeneous mass from the pile.

The compacted pile of sheets is then turned over on its side and sliced into new sheets, between 3 - 6 mm. usually, depending upon the requirements. The direction of cut is then at right angles to the plane of the original sheets. This produces the colour patterns which are characteristic of the sliced acetate.

The sliced acetate sheets have then to be conditioned for a period of several days at a fixed temperature to remove the original solvent. They are then ready for depatch and use.

The sliced acetate has a limited range of colours, the material slowly perishes in time and is affected by body acids (although not so readily as nitrate). These acids attack the molucular structure of the whole material as it is porous to a certain extent.

In order to produce extruded acetate slabs for spectacle frame production, the cellulose acetate in granular form incorporating suitable plasticiser is heated in a cylinder until molten, and is then squeezed under pressure through a slit whose depth and width determines the thickness and width of the extruded sheet. The obvious advantage of this method is that the finished sheets are the correct thickness required for subsequent machining.

The material as it comes through the slit is supported and kept straight, and at the same time chilled to produce the extruded material of infinite length. For convenience the extrusion is cut to a previously determined length as it leaves the cooling tank.

Colour effects in extruded material are produced by squeezing into the slit materials of different colours heated in different cylinders. The range of colours is much better than heretofore and is almost as good as the acrylic resins in this respect.

Extruded acetate is very much harder than sliced acetate and when polished has a surface film which is almost impervious to body acids. This obviously presents many and distinct advantages. In spite of this fact, it is very resilient and will sustain much bending and manipulation —surprisingly so. However, whilst much better than previously, even extruded acetate is not completely trouble-free and will in time perish like all plastics materials. This material is manufactured under various trade names such as "Acrylite", "Bexoid", "Rocel", etc.

Perspex has one serious drawback as compared with the cellulose materials, and that is that it is rather brittle. A sudden blow will fracture it. To compensate for this, it is lighter in weight, very much less affected by chemical action, and can take a beautiful range of colours which obviously creates a considerable source of attraction for ladies' frames. The temperature at which the frame is capable of having its shape altered is much higher than with nitrate or acetate. Consequently once it is adjusted to a certain shape and position by the optician, it will alter but little so maintaining the correct fitting on the patient's face. The cellulose materials all tend to warp in use—sliced acetate worst, extruded acetate next and nitrate least. However, none of them is as good as perspex or tortoiseshell in this respect.

All manufacturers carry out considerable research into this question of the quality of different materials for spectacle frame use. One British manufacturer made a number of frames from sliced acetate, nitrate, extruded acetate and perspex. They were then sent to South Africa where for many months they were placed on a roof-top. There is a considerable temperature and climatic range on the High Veldt, very hot by day and very cold by night. They were therefore subject alternately to conditions varying from scorching sun to frost, with the usual weather hazards of rain, hail, ice, etc. After this time, these frames were then tested to destruction, and extruded acetate proved from all points of view to be the most satisfactory.

This example of enquiry into the physical properties of plastics that are used for spectacle manufacturing, is quoted to show how research is constantly being applied to materials used for this purpose. Undoubtedly in the years to come, further development in the plastics industry will bring other materials to the fore.

Mention has been made throughout several of the preceding paragraphs to chemical action, body acids, etc. It is as well to bear in mind that probably the most important quality of any material used for spectacle manufacturing is that it must be chemically inert. It must come into contact with the skin and it must produce no deleterious affect. The number of materials which possess this property is very limited.

It is not easy to describe in a book the vast range of colours that is available in modern plastics materials, nor to convey by the printed word the visual impression which many frames made in perspex or extruded acetate, or as "combination" metal/plastics frames, are capable of giving. They must be seen to be appreciated.

Spectacle frame manufacturers are usually well aware of the cosmetic appeal of nicely styled and designed frames. Opticians should also be aware of this appeal, and should usually try and present the most attractive and modern frame styles.

(c) METALS. Steel has been used in the past for manufacturing spectacle frames, but for all practical purposes, is no longer used.

Nickel silver (also known as German silver) and pure nickel are both widely used, and both of these may be obtained gold-clad, or G.F. (gold-filled) as it is more generally known. G.F. material is also known as R.G. (rolled gold) but strictly speaking this is a different process. Base metals of beryllium copper may also be gold clad, but these are not so widely used in the manufacture of spectacle frames owing to difficulties in working them, particularly cold working.

Various techniques are used to process these metals, the greatest contrast being between the nickel silver and G.F. types. The nickel silver may be treated differently from the G.F. mainly because it is a common material throughout. It may therefore be machined or blanked. These processes cannot be carried out on G.F. as it is essential that the gold surface must remain unbroken except where one part will eventually be joined to another. An example of this may be found where the ends of a bridge will be eventually soldered to the eyewire. Parts made from gold-clad material can therefore only be formed by operations known as coining, striking, crimping and bending.

One of the most important factors governing the popularity of a frame is its rigidity or ability to hold its alignment. With non-ferrous metals, apart from using a heavy cross-section, strength can only be obtained by work hardening, that is by employing operations that move the molecular construction of the material thereby giving extra rigidity.

Raw material may be obtained from the manufacturers in various conditions specified by hardness numbers, which are determined by machine testing using depth-of-penetration methods. It may also be obtained in different sections usually in coils. If joints are to be made, for instance, the section would be rectangular, and if G.F., the gold cladding would appear on three sides of the nickel silver base.

When forming the joints, the G.F. material is processed in dies with highly polished faces so that the gold skin is drawn around the end. Various operations have to be carried out to achieve the shapes required, and this results in the material becoming very hard. So before the last operations are carried out, an annealing operation has to be performed to bring the parts back into a state capable of being worked on still further. In order that this may be done satisfactorily, the gold must be protected, so the parts are coated with a protective solution. They are then inserted in an electric furnace and raised to 680°C for a predetermined length of time to allow the heat to penetrate to the centre of the batch. After removal, the parts are water-cooled and cleaned, and the remaining operations carried out.

Great care must be exercised whilst soldering metal parts because to allow unrestricted heat flow along a material will alter its hardness. So a system of electric resistance soldering is employed, and clamps are used on the work which expose only a very small portion, thus allowing only localized heating to take place.

In an average metal frame, over 100 operations have to be performed before a complete frame is produced.

British Standards have been issued covering two aspects of metal frame manufacture, or parts made of metal used in frame manufacture. These are B.S. 3172 covering screw threads, whilst B.S. 3462 is a specification for metal spectacle frames and outlines various tests to which a frame should be subjected.

1.4. Experience

Essentially the topic of spectacle frames and materials is a very practical one, and nothing can take the place of experience in this context. The optician or student is always urged therefore at all times to enlarge his horizon as much as possible. He should make every endeavour to familiarize himself with each individual frame, its range of measurements and colours, the material (or materials) in its construction, its method of manufacture, the standards applied to it, and so on.

Detailed instruction on frame styles and measurements should be given to optical students. This is as important in the finished spectacles as the theory of optics, ophthalmic lenses, visual optics, and related matters. The optician who is unable to relate his technical "know-how" to accurate frame fitting is at a serious disadvantage, and his patients will achieve little benefit from a poorly fitted frame. More than this, they may be deriving unwanted optical effects due to displaced optical centres of lenses, wrong effectivity at the cornea, etc., to say nothing of the discomfort involved. This is a serious criticism and merits serious consideration.

1.5. Classification of Frame Patterns

Whilst the development of modern plastics materials has made the variety for spectacle frames quite bewildering, at the same time, there are several basic patterns into which these frames may conveniently be classified. This classification will be followed throughout this book for the purpose of describing the techniques of frame fitting.

This classification is as follows:-

(i) Pad bridge (both plastics, metal and combination).

(ii) Regular bridge.

(iii) Half-eye.

(iv) Supra.

1.6. Compromise of Interest between Patient and Optician

It is to be noted at this stage that there is sometimes a clash of interests between the optician's and/or patient's requirements for frames and lenses. For example, a person may request a very large size frame with, say, a 60 mm. round eye. However, the maximum size lens blank commercially made may be only 52 mm., or the production of this large size may entail a thick and heavy lens. So a compromise must be effected, which will obviously have to depend upon the circumstances of the particular case.

This necessity for compromise between what is desirable and what is technically possible; or between the optician and the spectacle wearer, arises very frequently in practice, so much so that this point will be referred to repeatedly in later chapters.

CHAPTER II

SYSTEMS OF MEASUREMENT

2.1. British Standards

2.1A. In 1960, British Standard No. B.S. 3199 was published by the British Standards Institution on the "Measurement of Spectacles". In 1962, a further standard, B.S. 3521 on the "Glossary of Terms relating to Ophthalmic Lenses and Spectacle Frames" was published. This latter is much more detailed in some of its information than the former, and of course relates to many matters which are not our immediate concern in this book.

2.1B. The relevant parts of B.S. 3199 are reproduced as an appendix to this chapter, and the reader is referred to it at this stage. It will be noted that most if not all the terms in use in frame manufacturing (except colloquial ones or those whose meaning is ambiguous or otherwise not clear) are included. Many of the terms need much more explanation and illustration than is provided in this necessarily brief schedule. Such for example are the references to the datum lens size and boxed lens size. Most of the rest of this chapter is devoted to a discussion about these two systems of measurement—the datum system and the boxed lens system.

2.1C. It has not been deemed necessary to define and explain most of the other terms in use in frame making and measuring, and where these terms are not explained in the text of this book, they are taken as being defined in B.S. 3199.

2.2. Systems in use in Gt. Britain and in Foreign Countries

There are two major systems of lens measurement (and of frame measurement to fit the lenses) in use throughout the world, being the DATUM SYSTEM as used in Gt. Britain and many other countries, and the BOX SYSTEM as used partly on the Continent of Europe and in

10

the U.S.A. Prior to the mid-1930s or thereabouts, there was a great deal of confusion due to the advent of upswept shapes which could no longer be measured by the previously accepted standards. The introduction of the datum system solved a great deal of this confusion, and has also been applied successfully to the further development of the supra style. However half-eye lens shapes are more usually measured by the box system.

This however does not end the subject, for many frame manufacturing companies have their own standards, and details are usually published by them of the basis of their systems of measurements.

2.3. The Datum System

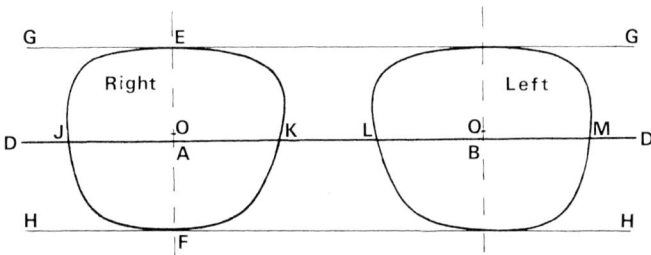

Fig. 2.1. Two symmetrically placed lens shapes, showing the position of the datum line DD.

Referring to Fig. 2.1. above, the datum line DD is the line half-way between the top and bottom horizontal tangents GG and HH to the lenses at their highest and lowest points. **Note particularly** that the tangents indicated by the lines GG and HH, are the tangents to the **lenses** not to the frames. If the frame is, say, a round or regular oval and the material of the same thickness top and bottom, then the mid-points of the tangents to the lenses and those to the frames will coincide. But if the frame shape

11

is upswept or has rims of varying thickness, or if it is supra, then it is the tangents to the top and bottom of the **lenses** that must be used to determine the datum line. This must be strictly understood to avoid a constant source of confusion.

The datum line DD is the basis of most measurements in the vertical plane of a spectacle front, particularly lens sizes and bridge measurements.

The points A and B midway between the horizontal extremities J – K and L – M of the right and left lenses respectively, are the datum centres. The distance AB is the datum centre distance. Due to long practice however and the continuation of some of the uncertainty of previous years, the datum centre distance is also known as the frame P.D., geometrical P.D., or the frame centre (F.C.) distance. (P.D. in this context refers to the pupillary distance, more strictly the inter-pupillary distance, see Ch. 3).

When a lens size is quoted by two measurements, viz. 44 mm. $\times$ 40 mm. or 44×40, these are the horizontal distance JK (the datum length) and the vertical distance EF (the mid-datum depth), both passing through the datum centre A. The difference between the two measurements, viz. 4 mm. as quoted above, is the shape difference. A lens size of 3 or 4 difference will be one of a deep shape; a lens size of say 10 difference will represent a shallow shape.

Lenses may of course be edged or glazed to various different kinds of frames or mounts. Consequently, the lenses may be bevel-edged, flat-edged, grooved or otherwise finished. In all cases, however, it is the highest point of the lens that is understood by the positions of the tangents GG and HH, and by the positions of J and K.

In any particular frame style, the shape difference will be established already, and thus it is only necessary to refer to the horizontal datum length, e.g. 44 Mirage; the fact that it is a "Mirage" shape automatically means that it must be 5 difference.

In addition to the horizontal and vertical lens sizes, there is one other important point on a lens which is shown as O in Fig. 2.1. This is the standard optical centre position, and is the position on the lens where the optical centre is to lie, provided there is no prism or decentration. In fact O always lies on the vertical through the datum centre, but its vertical position will depend on the Prescription House, some placing it on datum, most at $1\frac{1}{2}$ mm. above datum, and some even 2 mm. or 3 mm. above datum. The Prescription House should specify the standard optical centre position in its technical publications. In the event of horizontal prism or decentration, O will be moved parallel to DD, so that it may be decentred 5 mm. in for example, but will still be at the same horizontal height above DD.

2.4. The Box System

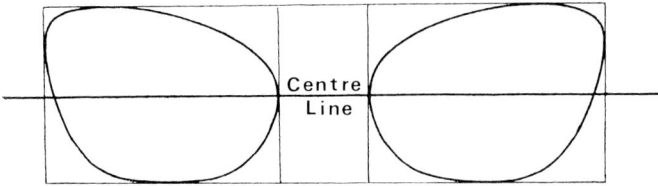

Fig. 2.2. Two symmetrically placed lens shapes, showing the position of the centre line.

In the box system, the horizontal and vertical tangents to the lenses form the boxed lens size. Half-way between the top and bottom tangents is the boxed lens size centre line. This is the line (corresponding to the datum line in the datum system) from which most measurements are taken—particularly bridge heights and spread, etc.

2.5. Frame fitting relative to Datum Line

The datum line is a line relative to the lens shape, and by symmetry to the two lenses mounted together in a frame. Since the normal practice in the optical world is to make a frame first (the lens shape of which is that of the required finished glazed lens), and then glaze the lenses to fit, it is obvious that the datum line therefore is a line relative to the frame, but not, it must be emphasized, mid-way between top and bottom tangents to the frame. The special case of the supra, where there is no lower rim to the frame, will be dealt with later (See ¶4.9 and ¶5.5.).

13

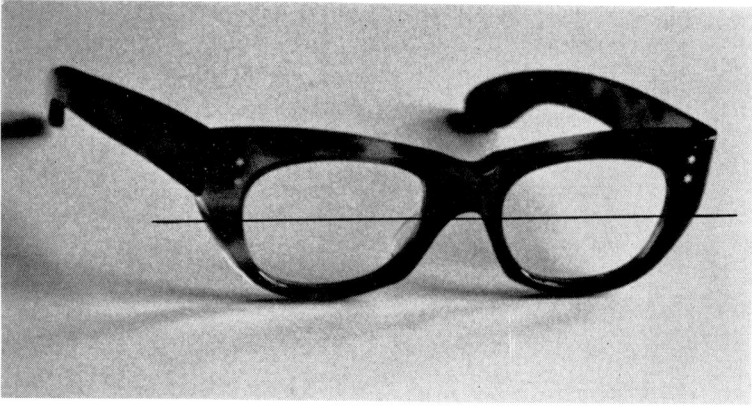

Fig. 2.3. Frame showing position of datum line.

Fig. 2.3 shows a frame with the datum line marked on it. Fig. 2.4a shows the same frame on a person in what might be loosely termed a "normal" or average position. Fig. 2.4b shows the same frame fitted on a person who holds the head high. This is typical of a person who has a very upright stance. Fig. 2.4c shows the same frame fitted on a person with the head held down. This is typical of a person who stoops, is very round-shouldered, or perhaps has a physical deformity.

To emphasize the point, the same subject has been shown in each position. It will be noted that the datum line, which is in a fixed position on the frame, is certainly not fixed on the subject. In Fig. 2.4a, the datum line passes about 1 mm. below the pupil's lower edge; or allowing an average size of 4 mm. for the pupil, about 3 mm. below the pupil centre. In Fig. 2.4b, the datum line passes about 1 mm. above the pupil centre, or 4 mm. higher than in Fig. 2.4a. In Fig. 2.4c, the datum line passes about 7 mm. below the pupil centre, or 4 mm. lower than in Fig. 2.4a.

2.6. Important Note about Datum Line

It should therefore be borne in mind that when referring to the datum line (or the boxed lens size centre line), that it is the frame or lens shape that is meant, and not the person on whom the spectacles have to be fitted. Students in particular seem to have difficulty in relating this fundamental concept to their fitting techniques.

14

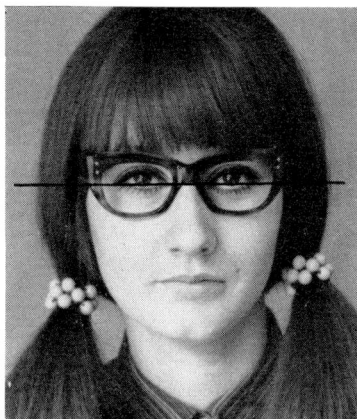

Fig. 2.4a. Frame on face: head in normal position.

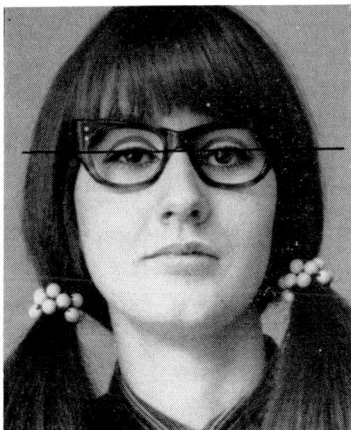

Fig. 2.4b. Frame on face: head held high.

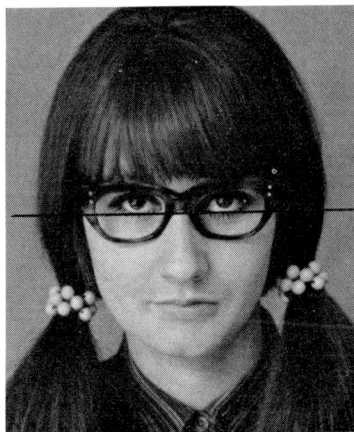

Fig. 2.4c. Frame on face: head held down.

2.7. Position of Datum Line of Frame Relative to Persons' Eyes

Referring therefore to Fig. 2.4a, it is generally accepted that the datum line should be positioned just below the lower edge of the pupil in normal cases. The optical centre of the lens is usually glazed $1\frac{1}{2}$ mm. or 2 mm. above the datum centre position (assuming no decentration), which is the standard optical centre position (see also B.S. 3199). For bifocals, it is usual to position the segment top 2 mm. below the datum line in the absence of any other information or requirements. For Varilux or similar graduated lenses, it is often necessary to position the start of the progression above datum by 2 mm. or 3 mm. However the positioning of bifocals and multifocals of all types (including Varilux) needs considerable further discussion (see ¶3.9).

One final comment should be inserted here to show the difference between principle and practice. The injuction to the optician is to position the datum line of the frame about 3 mm. below the centre of the pupil in normal cases with the eyes looking ahead. However it will be found in practice that most people hold their heads down somewhat in use. Most of our lives are spent within the confines of rooms or looking into the near distance, and we have to look where we are walking. So the natural tendency is to hold the head tilted down somewhat. Also, most spectacle sides slip in use which permits the frame to drop down the nose a little from its initially (and ideally) fitted position. The result is that most people tend to look through points more nearly 5 mm. above the datum line, and in many cases even more.

2.8. "Normal" Position

From what has been said so far, it will be noted that to a large extent the secret of successful frame fitting depends on what may be defined as a "normal" or average position of the head of the subject when the frame is being fitted. This point having been raised will be dealt with at length during the next few chapters, but to a large extent this is a matter of judgment and experience on the part of the optician. His skill and practice which are gradually built up over a period of time by seeing and dealing with many hundreds or even thousands of patients, enable him to say from experience that a certain frame positioned in a certain way on a certain face held in a certain position, constitutes a "normal" situation for that particular set of circumstances. Another even more intangible factor in successful frame fitting lies in gaining the confidence of the patient. This matter will also be raised later.

APPENDIX

BRITISH STANDARD 3199

MEASUREMENT OF SPECTACLES

METHOD AND GLOSSARY

MEASUREMENT OF SPECTACLES
Method and Glossary

FOREWORD

The object of this British Standard is to define an acceptable system of spectacle measurement adapted to present-day requirements. The principal dimensions are based on the datum line, but provision has been made for certain additional dimensions derived from other concepts.

In the main, existing terminology has been retained, but a few changes have been thought desirable. It is thought that the new term ' datum centre ' will be found particularly useful. To prevent confusion, the terms ' geometrical centre ' and ' eyesize ' have been deliberately avoided.

The advent of new frame styles has rendered necessary a more precise definition of the principal reference plane and a new approach to certain dimensions such as ' length to bend '. As far as possible, however, accepted definitions which have hitherto occasioned no difficulties have been retained in their familiar form.

The standard includes definitions of a few dimensions which in practice are rarely specified but which have been included for the sake of completeness and to facilitate discussion of the principles of frame design and fitting; such measurements should be stated as will, however, taken in conjunction with the prescription and any dimensions published by the manufacturer, specify adequately the frame or spectacles. Recommended abbreviations are shown in parentheses.

It has now been found possible to define ' standard optical centre position ' more precisely than in B.S. 2738, ' Spectacle lenses '.

Attention is drawn to the fact that the height of a metal W-bridge is defined in accordance with the accepted method used for frames made of plastics materials.

Other British Standards relating to ophthalmic subjects include the following:

B.S. 2738. Spectacle lenses.
B.S. 3062. Spectacle lens materials.
B.S. 3162. Ophthalmic trial case lenses.
B.S. 3172. Screw threads of unified form for spectacle frames, including screwing taps and gauges.
B.S. 3186. Cellulose acetate sheet for spectacle frames.

SPECIFICATION

PART 1. METHOD OF MEASUREMENT OF SPECTACLES

SCOPE

1. This British Standard defines a system of spectacle measurement.

TERMS AND DEFINITIONS

2. The terms and definitions used for this system of spectacle measurement shall be as given in the Glossary (Part 2).

REFERENCE LINES AND PLANES

3. The frame or mount shall be considered as oriented so that the back plane of the front is vertical and as though worn on the face. Lens and spectacle measurements shall then be related to the following reference lines and planes:

a. Back plane of the front (see 4101).

b. Horizontal and vertical tangents to the lens shape (see 1101).

c. Datum line of lens (see 1102).

d. Datum line of frame or mount (see 4102).

MEASUREMENTS

4. *a.* All measurements and associated reference lines relating to lenses shall be taken to the edge of the lens, that is, to the peak of the bevel (if any).

b. Measurements shall be taken with the frame or mount opened or extended as in use.

c. All linear measurements shall be expressed in millimetres. Where a minus sign is prefixed to a dimension it shall be understood to mean that the measurement is downwards from the datum line or backwards from the back plane of the front, whichever is applicable.

d. Lens sizes shall be specified by numbers denoting the dimensions in millimetres, the horizontal dimension being invariably given first.

Examples:

40 × 36 signifies 40 mm long and 36 mm deep.

38 round signifies a round lens of 38 mm diameter.

STANDARD OPTICAL CENTRE POSITION

5. The standard optical centre position shall invariably be located on a vertical line passing through the datum centre (see 1103). The horizontal distance

19

between the right and left in a pair of lenses will, therefore, be equal to the datum centre distance (see 4106).

The height of the standard optical centre position for any given lens shape shall be as published by the manufacturer, but in the absence of any such publication the standard optical centre position shall be the datum centre.

NOTE. The height of the standard optical centre position as defined above may not apply to half-eye and similar shapes nor to bifocal and multifocal lenses, but manufacturers are recommended to publish the rules they apply in the absence of specific instructions regarding centration.

DECENTRATIONS

6. *a.* Horizontal decentrations shall be specified as a distance from the standard optical centre position (with reference to a given frame or mount) or by stating the desired centration distance (see 2103) in which case any necessary decentration shall be equally divided between the two lenses.

b. Vertical decentrations shall be specified as a distance above or below the standard optical centre position.

PART 2. GLOSSARY OF TERMS

SECTION ONE: LENS DIMENSIONS AND LENS TERMS

No.	Term	Definition
1101	**Lens shape**	The outline of the lens periphery with the nasal side and the horizontal indicated.
1102	**Datum line of lens** (dat L)	The line mid-way between, and parallel to, the horizontal tangents to the lens shape at its highest and lowest points (see Fig. 1).
1103	**Datum centre** (dat C)	The mid-point of that part of the datum line which is bounded by the lens shape (see Fig. 2).
1104	**Datum lens size**	The horizontal and vertical dimensions of the lens, measured through the datum centre (see Fig. 2). These dimensions may be referred to as datum length and mid-datum depth respectively (also see Part 1, Clause 4 d).
1105	**Boxed lens size**	The size of the rectangle containing the lens shape and formed by the horizontal and vertical tangents to the lens shape (see Fig. 3) (also see Part 1, Clause 4 d). This specification may be given in addition to the datum lens size.
		NOTE. In the case of half-eye and similar shapes, the boxed lens size should be specified instead of the datum lens size.
1106	**Shape difference**	The difference in millimetres between the horizontal and vertical dimensions of the lens, with reference to a specified system of lens size measurement (see 1104 and 1105).
		NOTE. This should be expressed as in the examples: ' Shape 4 dat ' or ' Shape 6 boxed '. In the absence of any indication, the datum lens size will be assumed.

SECTION TWO: OPTICAL CENTRATION

2101	**Standard optical centre position**	A reference point peculiar to each lens shape (see Part 1, Clause 5). The optical centre is located at this point in the absence of instructions to the contrary, any prescribed prisms having first been neutralized.
2102	**Centration point (CP)**	The point at which the optical centre is to be located in the absence of prescribed prism or after any prescribed prism has been neutralized.
2103	**Centration distance** (CD)	The horizontal distance between the right and left centration points.
		NOTE. If an inter-pupillary distance only is stated, this should be taken to be the centration distance.
2104	**Decentration** (dec)	A displacement, horizontal and/or vertical, of the centration point from the standard optical centre position.

21

No.	Term	Definition
2105	**Bodily decentration**	A term used in reference to lenticulars to indicate that the decentration applies to the lenticular aperture as well as to the centration point.

NOTE. This term is also applied to bifocals to indicate a displacement of both distance and near portions.

SECTION THREE: BIFOCAL AND MULTIFOCAL SEGMENT DIMENSIONS AND TERMS

No.	Term	Definition
3101	**Segment diameter**	The diameter of the circle of which the boundary of the finished segment forms a part (see Fig. 4, dimensions).
3102	**Segment depth**	The vertical extent, measured through the segment top or the segment bottom whichever applies (see 3107 and 3110), of a segment which nowhere extends to the periphery of the lens (see Fig. 4c, dimension v).
3103	**Segment size**	A specification consisting of segment diameter and segment depth.
3104	**Geometrical inset** (G in)	The distance between vertical lines through the distance centration point and the mid-point of the segment diameter (see Fig. 5, dimension i).
3105	**Optical inset** (O in)	The horizontal displacement of the near or intermediate optical centre relative to the distance optical centre, prescribed prisms being neutralized in all portions.
3106	**Near visual point** (NVP)	An assumed position of the point at which the visual axis cuts the back surface of the lens in near vision, used as a reference point for calculating prismatic effects.
3107	**Segment top**	(Applicable only to a segment in the lower portion of the lens)

a. The point of contact of the curve forming the upper boundary (imaginary if broken by a re-entrant arc) of the segment with its horizontal tangent (see Figs. 4*a* and 4*b*, point T), or

b. In the case of a straight-topped segment the mid-point of the straight top (see Fig. 4*c*, point T).

No.	Term	Definition
3108	**Segment top position**	The vertical distance of the segment top above or below the datum line. This dimension is frequently given as in the example: ' Segment 2 below datum '.

NOTE. In the absence of instructions to the contrary, this dimension will be assumed to apply to the highest segment of a multifocal lens.

No.	Term	Definition
3109	**Segment height**	The vertical distance of the segment top above the horizontal tangent to the lens periphery at its lowest point (see Fig. 4, dimension u) (also see Note to 3108).

No.	Term	Definition
3110	**Segment bottom**	(Applicable only to a segment in the upper portion of the lens) a. The point of contact of the curve forming the lower boundary of the segment with its horizontal tangent, or b. In the case of a straight-bottomed segment, the mid-point of the straight bottom.
3111	**Segment bottom position**	The vertical distance of the segment bottom above or below the datum line.

SECTION FOUR: DIMENSIONS AND TERMS APPLYING TO FRONTS GENERALLY

4101	**Back plane of the front**	The surface of the frame or mount nearer to the eyes. It coincides with the back surface of the eyerims or, in rimless mounts having a separate bridge, with the back plane of the clamps or straps. When the eyerims do not lie substantially in one plane, and in the case of rimless brow-bar and similar mounts, the back plane of the front is the plane containing symmetrical small parts of both eyerims or both brow-bars immediately adjacent to the bridge.
4102	**Datum line of frame or mount** (dat L)	The line coincident with the datum lines of the lenses (see Fig. 6, line DD). NOTE 1. In the case of a frame or mount in which the datum lines of the lenses are not continuous, one lens being higher than the other, it should be clearly stated to which of these datum lines given measurements refer. NOTE 2. When using a frame measuring rule in which the frame or mount is positioned by reference to the outside of the eyerims, due allowance should be made if the eyerims are of different thickness at the top and the bottom.
4103	**Lens size of frame or mount**	The size of the lenses that the frame or mount is designed to hold.
4104	**Distance between lenses** (DBL)	The horizontal distance, measured along the datum line between the nasal edges of the lenses (see Fig. 6, dimension d).
4105	**Minimum between lenses** (MBL)	The horizontal distance between the vertical tangents to the nasal edges of the lens shapes (see Fig. 6, dimension m).
4106	**Datum centre distance** (dat CD)	The horizontal distance between the right and left datum centres (see Fig. 6, dimension c). NOTE. Datum centre distance = Datum length of lens + Distance between lenses.
4107	**Frontal width** (FW)	The horizontal distance between the centres of the dowel pins or dowel screws.
4108	**Height of bridge** (ht)	The vertical distance from the datum line to the mid-point of the lower edge of the bridge (see Fig. 7 and Part 1, Clause 4 c).

23

No.	Term	Definition
4109	Projection (or inset) of bridge (proj)	The minimum horizontal distance from the back plane of the front to the centre of the back of the bridge (see Figs. 8 and 9 and Part 1, Clause 4 c).
4110	Angle of crest (AC)	Of a W-bridge (metal) or regular bridge (plastics), the angle in a vertical plane between a line tangential to the bearing surface at its centre and the back plane of the front (see Fig. 10). This measurement, if applied to a pad bridge, should be taken from the line approximating to the back surface of the bar in a central section.

SECTION FIVE: DIMENSIONS PECULIAR TO W AND REGULAR BRIDGES

1. W-BRIDGES (METAL)

5101	Base of bridge (B)	The distance between the extremities of the bearing surface (see Fig. 11, dimension j).
5102	Depth of bridge (D)	The distance, measured in the plane of the arch, between the centre of the bearing surface of the crest and the line joining the extremities of the bearing surface (see Fig. 11, dimension k).
5103	Apical radius (AR)	The radius of the circle, in the plane of the arch, which fits the bearing surface of the crest (see Fig. 11, dimension r).

2. REGULAR BRIDGES (PLASTICS MATERIALS)

5201	Base and depth of bridge	The base is the horizontal distance between the nasal surfaces of the eyerims, measured at a stated depth below the mid-point of the lower edge of the bridge.
		NOTE. This dimension should always be expressed as in the example ' base 19 at 10 below crest ' (see Fig. 12) to emphasize that the measurement is taken as in this definition and not relative to the datum line.
5202	Apical radius (AR)	The radius of the arc forming the lower edge of the bridge viewed perpendicularly to the back plane of the front (see Fig. 13).

SECTION SIX: DIMENSIONS PECULIAR TO PAD BRIDGES

1. GENERAL

6101	Distance between rims (DBR)	The horizontal distance between the nasal edges of the eyerims, measured and stated along the datum line (see Fig. 6, dimension e) or at any specified level above or below the datum line. Examples: (i) DBR 16 dat. (ii) DBR 20 at 10 below dat.
6102	Pad centre	Of fixed pads, the point on the bearing surface equidistant from its top and bottom, and front and back, edges. Of rocking pads, the point on the bearing surface opposite the point of attachment of the pad.
6103	Pad plane	A plane approximating to the bearing surface of the pad.

No.	Term	Definition
6104	Vertical angle of pad	The angle between the back plane of the front and the long axis of the pad projected on a vertical plane at right angles to the back plane of the front. This is the apparent angle between the long axis of the pad and the back plane of the front, viewed horizontally along this plane (see Fig. 14).
		NOTE. Unless otherwise specified, this angle will be regarded as bringing the top of the pad relatively backwards, as in Fig. 14.
6105	Frontal angle of pad	The angle between the vertical and the line of intersection of the pad plane with the back plane of the front (see Fig. 15, angle A).
6106	Splay angle of pad	The angle between the pad plane and a normal to the back plane of the front (see Fig. 15, angle B).

2. PADS MOUNTED ON ARMS

6201	Height of pad centre (pad ht)	The vertical distance from the datum line to the pad centre (see Part 1, Clause 4 c).
6202	Distance between pad centres (DBP)	The horizontal distance between the two pad centres.
6203	Inset of pad centre	The horizontal distance from the back plane of the front to the pad centre.

3. PADS ATTACHED DIRECTLY TO EYERIMS

6301	Height of pad top (pad ht)	The vertical distance from the datum line to the highest point of the pad (see Part 1, Clause 4 c).
6302	Distance between pad tops	The horizontal distance between the tops of the pads.
6303	Width of pad	The maximum width of the pad surface, measured from the back of the eyerim.

SECTION SEVEN: DIMENSIONS AND TERMS RELATING TO JOINTS AND SIDES

1. GENERAL

7101	Joint height (jt ht)	The distance from the datum line to the horizontal plane through the centre of the joint.
7102	Joint size (jt)	The overall axial length of the charniers.
7103	Joint angle	The vertical angle, inherent in the construction of a joint, which contributes to the angle of side (see 7107).
7104	Ear point	a. Of a hockey-end side, the mid-point of the arc of contact between the bend of the side and the circle which fits it (see Fig. 16, point E).
		b. Of a curl-side, the point on the lower edge of the side at the beginning of the curl (see Fig. 21, point E).
		c. Of a straight side, the point on the lower edge of the side which is assumed to make contact with the top of the ear.

25

No.	Term	Definition
7105	**Dowel point**	The centre of the bottom of the dowel hole (see Figs. 16 and 21, point Q).
7106	**Line of the side**	The straight line through the dowel point and the ear point (see Figs. 16 and 21, line SS). NOTE. In the case of short straight sides, the line of the side shall be taken to be the lower edge of the side.
7107	**Angle of side**	The vertical angle between a normal to the back plane of the front and the line of the side when opened (see Fig. 16, angle C). NOTE. Unless otherwise specified the angle of the side is downwards from the normal to the back plane of the front at the middle of the joint.
7108	**Let-back of side**	The horizontal angle between the inner surface of the fully opened side, adjacent to the joint, and a normal to the back plane of the front (see Fig. 17, angle D).
7109	**Distance between sides (DBS at . . .)**	The distance between the inner surfaces of the fully opened sides at any specified position.
7110	**Temple width (TW)**	The distance between sides 25 mm behind the back plane of the front (see Fig. 17, dimension t).
7111	**Swept-back lug**	A swept-back extension of the front, to which the side is attached.
7112	**Lug point**	(Applicable only to swept-back lugs.) A point on the back surface of the lug where it begins its backward sweep, approximately level with the dowel point (see Fig. 18, point L).

2. DROP-END SIDES

No.	Term	Definition
7201	**Length to bend (TB)**	The distance between the dowel point and the ear point.
7202	**Front to bend (FTB)**	The distance between the lug point and the ear point.
7203	**Length of drop**	The distance from the ear point to the extreme end of the side (see Fig. 19, dimension g).
7204	**Downward angle of drop**	The downward inclination of the drop from the line of the side, measured near the ear point and in the vertical plane containing the line of the side (see Fig. 19, angle F).
7205	**Inward angle of drop**	The inward inclination of the drop near the ear point from the vertical plane containing the line of the side (see Fig. 20).
7206	**Head width**	The distance between the sides at the ear points (see Fig. 17, dimension w).

3. CURL SIDES

No.	Term	Definition
7301	**Total length**	The overall length from the dowel point to the extreme end.
7302	**Length to tangent**	The distance from the dowel point to that tangent to the inner surface of the curl at rest which is perpendicular to the line of the side (see Fig. 21).

4. STRAIGHT SIDES

No.	Term	Definition
7401	**Length**	The distance from the dowel point to the extreme end, the side being flattened.

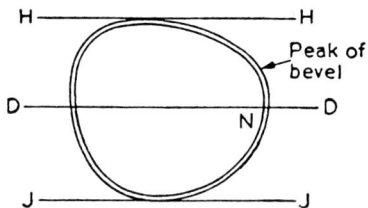

Fig. 1. Datum line of lens

HH, JJ = Horizontal tangents
DD = Datum line

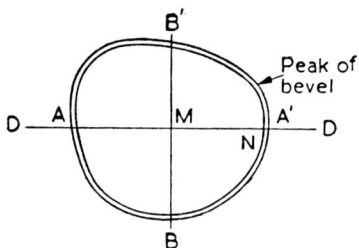

Fig. 2. Datum centre and lens size

DD = Datum line
AA′ = Datum length of lens
M = Datum centre (mid-point of AA
BB′ = Mid-datum depth of lens
(measured through M)

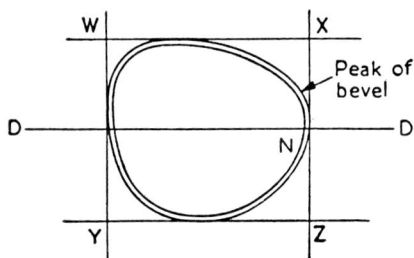

Fig. 3. Boxed lens size

DD = Datum line
WXYZ = Limiting rectangle defining boxed lens size

NOTE. In Figs. 1 to 5, N indicates the nasal side of the lens shape.

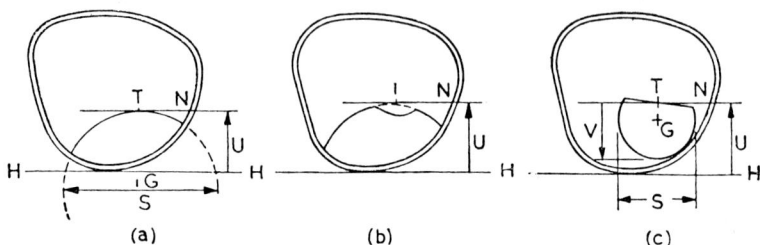

Fig. 4. Segment dimensions

HH = Horizontal tangent at lowest point on lens periphery
T = Segment top
G = Mid-point of segment diameter
s = Segment diameter
u = Segment height
v = Segment depth

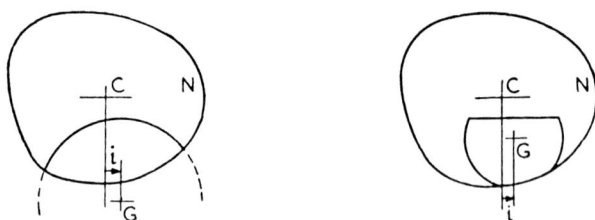

Fig. 5. Geometrical inset

C = Distance centration point
G = Mid-point of segment diameter
i = Geometrical inset

NOTE. In Figs. 1 to 5, N indicates the nasal side of the lens shape.

28

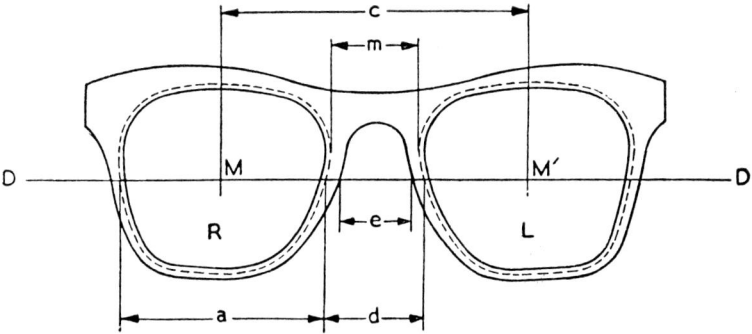

Fig. 6. Dimensions applying to fronts

The dotted curves represent peak of bevel or bottom of groove

DD = Datum line of frame	c = Datum centre distance
M = Datum centre of right lens	d = Distance between lenses
M′ = Datum centre of left lens	e = Distance between rims (dat)
a = Datum length of lens	m = Minimum between lenses

NOTE. c = a + d

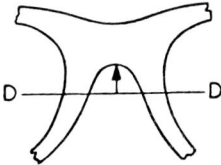

Fig. 7. Height of bridge
DD = Datum line

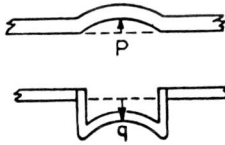

Fig. 8. projection (or inset) of bridge
p = Projection
q = Inset

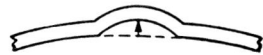

Fig. 9. Projection of bridge when eyerims do not lie substantially in a plane

29

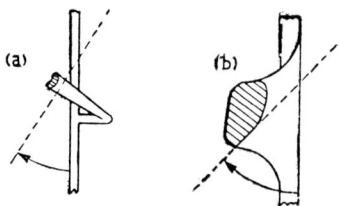

Fig. 10. Angle of crest
Diagram shows vertical section through centre
(a) W-bridge (metal)
(b) Regular bridge (plastics)

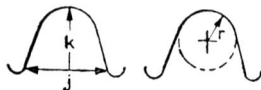

Fig. 11. Dimensions of W-bridge
Diagram shows central section in the plane of the arch
j = Base of bridge
k = Depth of bridge
r = Apical radius

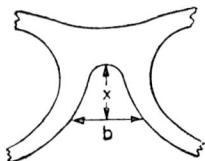

Fig. 12. Base and depth of regular bridge (plastics)
b = Base at depth x

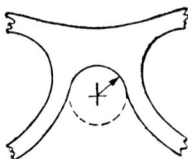

Fig. 13. Apical radius of regular bridge (plastics)

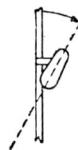

Fig. 14. Vertical angle of pad

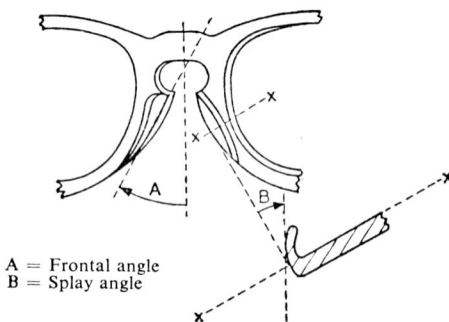

A = Frontal angle
B = Splay angle

Fig. 15. Pad angles

30

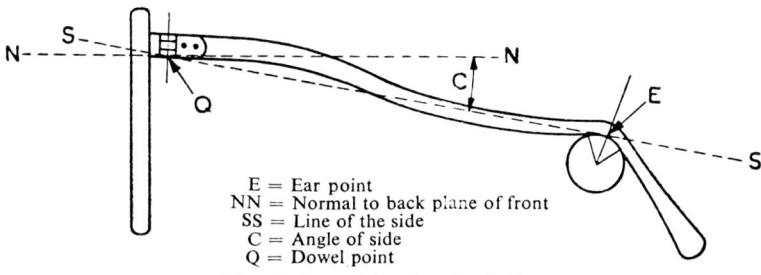

```
E  = Ear point
NN = Normal to back plane of front
SS = Line of the side
C  = Angle of side
Q  = Dowel point
```

Fig. 16. Ear point and angle of side

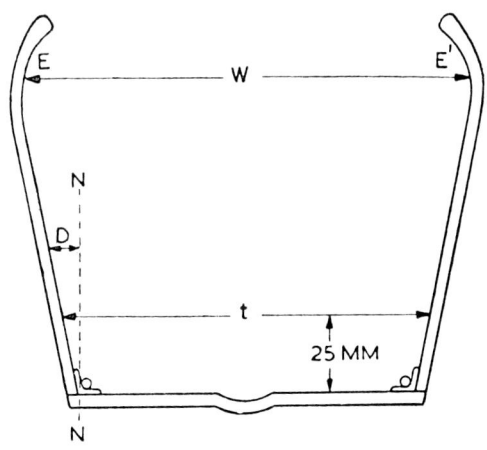

Fig. 17. Temple and head width: angle of let-back

```
E, E' = Ear points
NN = Normal to back plane of front
t  = Temple width
w  = Head width
D  = Angle of let-back
```

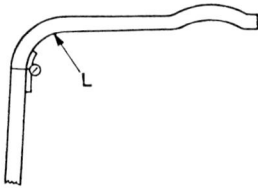

Fig. 18. Lug point (L)

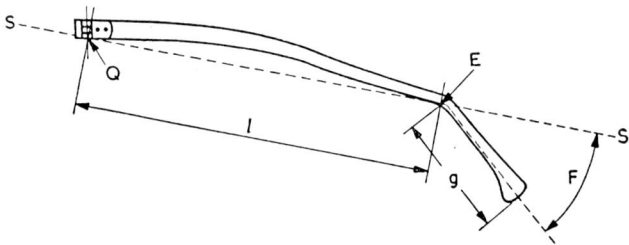

Fig. 19. Dimensions of drop-end sides

E = Ear point
SS = Line of the side
l = Length to bend
g = Length of drop
F = Downward angle of drop
Q = Dowel point

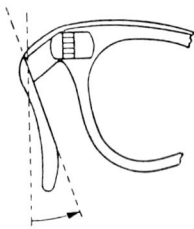

Vertical
Fig. 20. Inward angle of drop

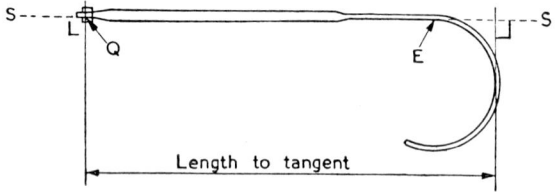

Length to tangent

Fig. 21. Length to tangent

32

CHAPTER III

P.D. AND EYE MEASUREMENTS

3.1. P.D. (inter-pupillary distance)

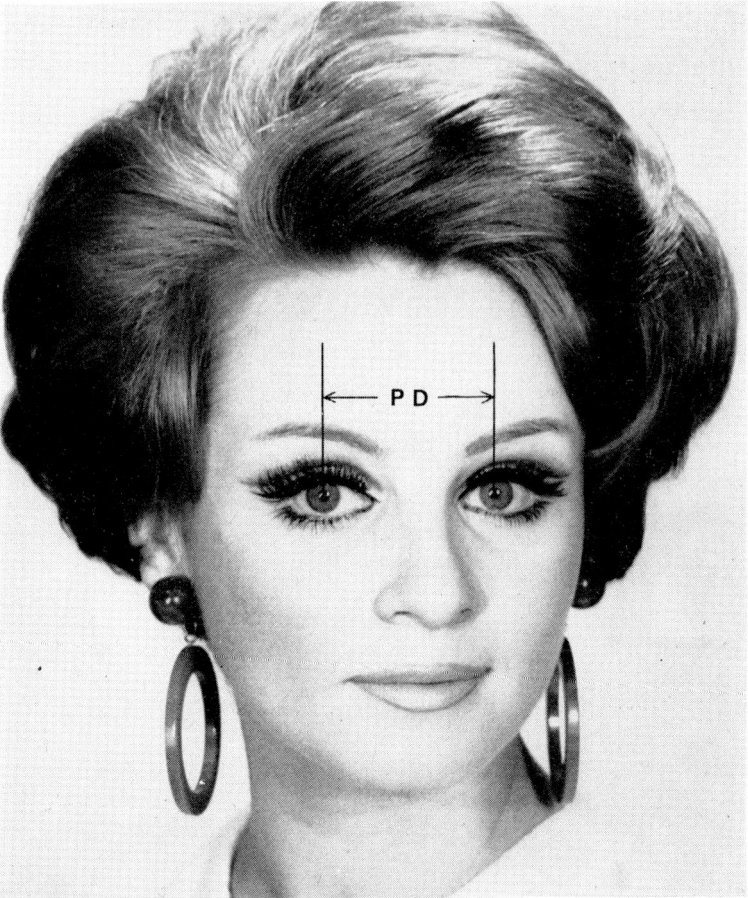

Fig. 3.1. P.D. (inter-pupillary distance)

33

The most important facial measurement that has to be determined is the inter-pupillary distance, usually known as the pupillary distance or P.D. for short. This is the distance apart horizontally of the centres of the two pupils. (Fig. 3.1).

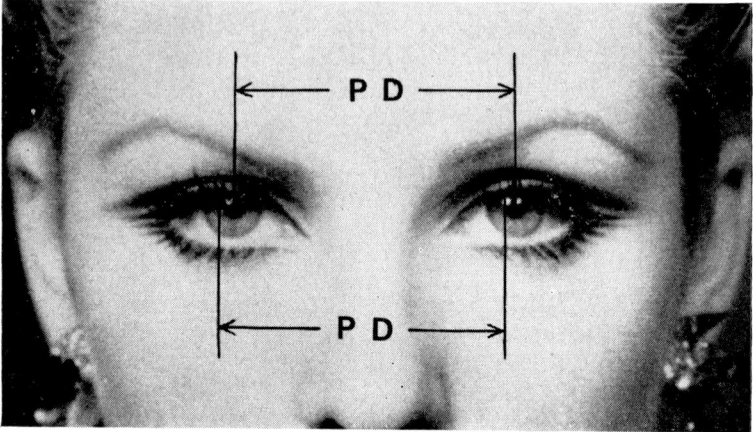

Fig. 3.2. P.D. is the distance apart of the centres of the pupils, or from the edge of one pupil to the corresponding edge of the other.

It will be apparent from Fig. 3.2 that providing the two pupils are symmetrical, a measurement from the temporal edge of the right pupil to the nasal edge of the left pupil, will give the same horizontal distance as the measurement from the right pupil centre to the left pupil centre. As the pupil is invariably black to the observer and about 4 mm. in diameter indoors (when partially dilated), it is difficult to determine by observation where its centre lies. A measurement from one edge of one pupil to the corresponding edge of the other pupil will therefore give the same result.

Various factors may prevent this method of determining the P.D. from being followed.
(i)   asymmetrical pupils.
(ii) dark irides.
(iii) squint or other physical displacement of one eye from a "normal" position.

3.1(i). Asymmetrical pupils
Where the two pupils are not of the same size or are not placed in the centres of the irides, no hard and fast rule can be laid down as to how the P.D. should be measured.

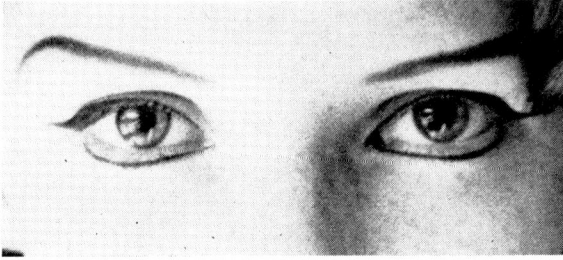

Fig. 3.3. Asymmetrical pupils showing the left pupil more dilated than the right.

This sort of situation may be encountered in a young person (Fig. 3.3 as illustrated) but is more usually encountered in uniocular aphakia. One eye or the other may have had an operation for removal of the crystalline lens following the development of a cataract.

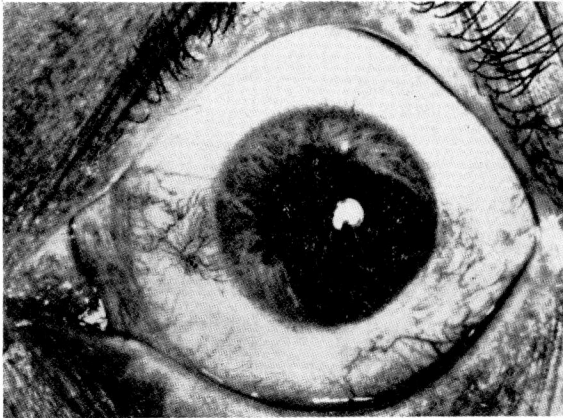

Fig. 3.4. An iridectomy operation has been performed on this eye, resulting in the removal of part of the iris.

If the eye has had an iridectomy operation performed on it, the asymmetry may be very irregular as illustrated in Fig. 3.4. The other eye, especially in an older person, may have a very small pupil.

Note: Uniocular — pertaining to one eye.

Aphakia — without a lens.

Iridectomy — an operation in which part of the iris is removed, generally to assist internal drainage of the eye.

Cataract — a condition in which the lens of the eye becomes opaque.

35

3.1 (ii). Dark irides

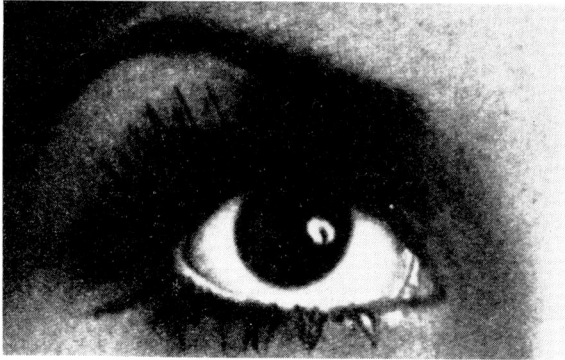

Fig. 3.5. Very dark iris.

In the dark-skinned races of mankind, there is a lot of pigmentation present in the iris which is often very dark brown. Particularly if the light is poor, it is difficult if not impossible to tell where the edge of the pupil lies (Fig. 3.5). In cases such as this therefore, the same method as shown in Fig. 3.2 may be applied, but measuring from the temporal edge of the right iris to the nasal edge of the left iris. Again care must be exercised to see that neither pupils nor irides are asymmetrical.

3.1(iii). Squint or other physical displacement of one eye from a "normal" position.

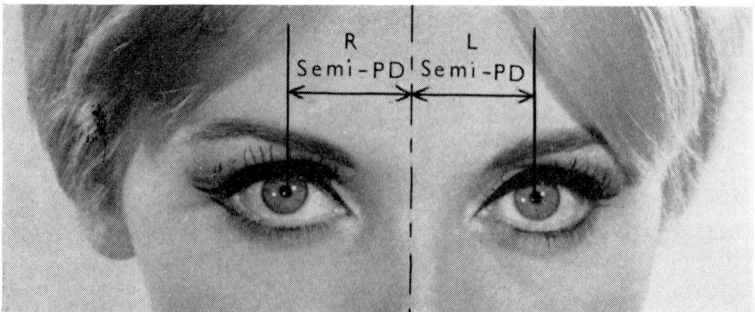

Fig. 3.6a. Right and left semi-P.Ds. are equal.

In Fig. 3.6a, the normal position is stated to be the situation where the right and left semi-P.D.s are equal, i.e. each eye is symmetrically disposed

36

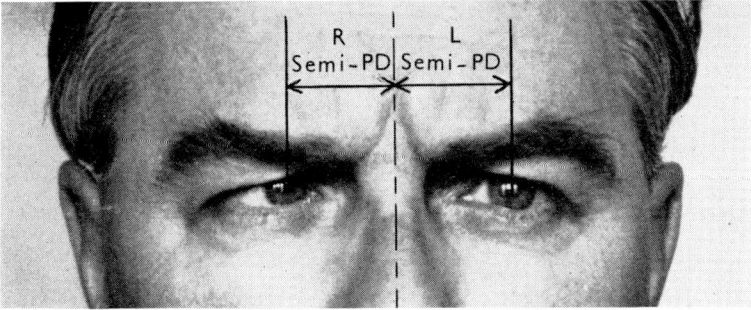

Fig. 3.6b. Right and left semi-P.Ds. are unequal: left greater than right.

on each side of the median line of the face. In Fig. 3.6b we have a situation where there is a squint of the right eye so that the left semi-P.D. is greater than the right semi-P.D. Possibly the right eye may be placed laterally nearer the nose, without squinting, but as far as we are concerned in this context, the result is the same, although the cause is different.

We should also explain what is meant by the median line of the face. Long practice uses this term a little loosely. What we mean is the vertical line passing midway through the bridge of the nose on a level with the eyes or a little below this level. Many persons have "broken" noses, the bridges of which may well be off-set from the median line of the face. Many persons have noses which appear to deviate from the vertical by a marked extent from bridge to tip.

The optician must use his judgement and experience. The median line must pass through the mid-point of the nose approximately where the spectacles are to rest. It is then for the optician to look carefully, and to try several spectacle frames on the subject if necessary, to determine whether there is any difference in the two semi-P.D. measurements.

3.2. Measurement of P.D.

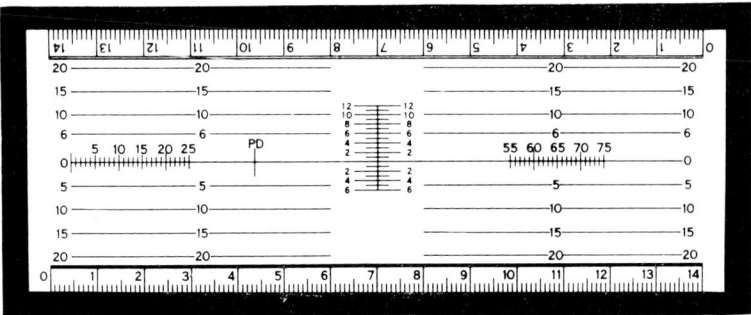

Fig. 3.7. Optical ruler.

37

The P.D. may be measured with an ivorine rule (white plastic) with black millimetre divisions marked on its edge. (Fig. 3.7).

There are a lot of other measurements marked on this rule, but we are concerned for the moment with the lower edge only.

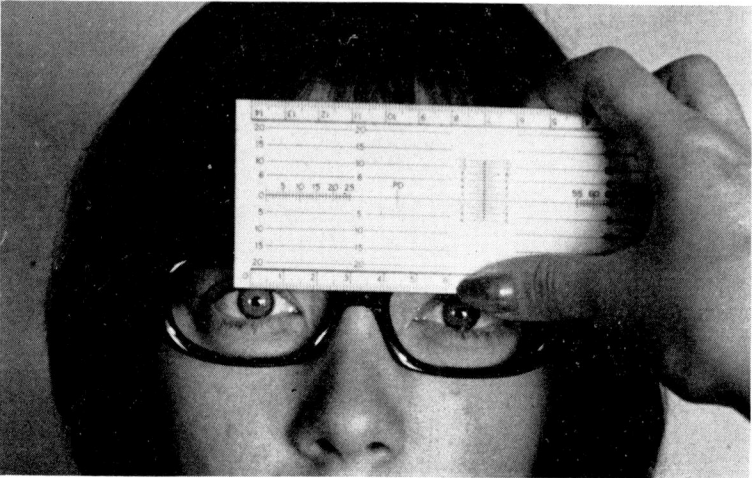

Fig. 3.8. Measurement of P.D. using optical ruler.

This figure (Fig. 3.8) shows how the measurement of P.D. is undertaken by a right-handed person.

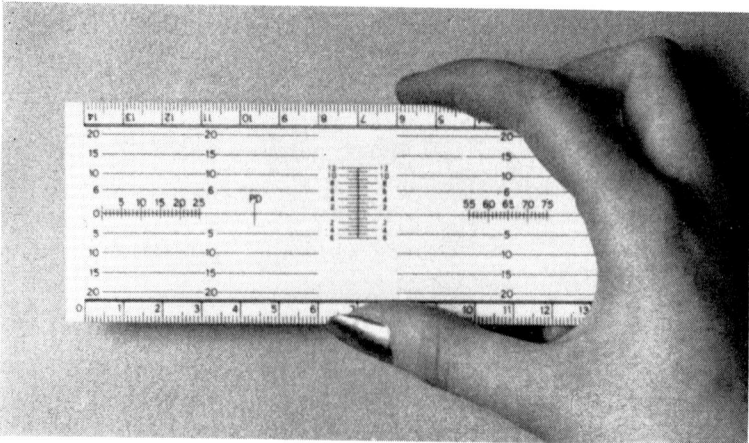

Fig. 3.9. Ruler removed from patient's face for easier observation.

The rule is held in the right hand, so that the four fingers grip the top and rest against the forehead. The thumb should be able to slide along the lower edge. The zero of the scale is held vertically above the temporal edge of the right pupil, and the thumb (held roughly at 60 mm. to start with) is moved horizontally to right or left until it comes to rest so that the nasal edge of the left pupil can just be seen. The rule is then removed with the thumb in this position, and the optician can see what measurement has been made. Fig. 3.9 shows the thumbnail resting against the 62 mm. scale division.

Care must be taken to see that the P.D. measured is that required for the purpose called for in the prescription, either distance or near (or such other as may be specifically required).

If the distance P.D. is required, the patient is directed to look into the left eye of the optician (or at a pencil held in front of the left eye) and the zero of the scale placed over the temporal edge of the right eye of the subject. The optician then directs the patient to look into his right eye (or moves the pencil across in front of the other eye). The patient's two eyes which have previously fixated upon the optician's left eye will now both move to fixate upon his right eye. The thumb is now moved quickly so that the nasal edge of the left pupil can just be seen. Again the P.D. is the measurement shown on the rule by the thumbnail.

The reason for this is three-fold: firstly the necessity to eliminate parallax; secondly the lack of comparision between the two semi-P.D. measurements (see also ¶3.5); and thirdly the necessity to reduce "wobble" due to shaky hands, attempts to avoid touching the patient, etc.

If the optician has a distant object at which he can direct his patient's view, then the measurement of the P.D. from the centre of one pupil to the centre of the other, will be correct. In the close confines of a room however, this is seldom the case, and alternative methods have to be adopted.

Parallax must be avoided. The patient's eyes, the rule and the optician's eyes must all be in line. Experience will teach the optician to hold his head and his rule so that this trouble is kept to a minimum. However, a great deal of practice is necessary, and checking and verification by other more experienced persons is required for a long time in the case of trainees. This is a surprizingly difficult technique to acquire and master properly.

If the near P.D. is required, then the patient is directed to look into one eye of the optician (or at a pencil or some other convenient point of fixation). It is important for the optician to position himself or his patient at the reading distance, say 30 – 40 cm. The distance apart of the pupils is then measured.

When the patient is asked to fixate upon a near point in front of him, he will obviously accommodate and converge. When one eye is occluded (as covering with the thumb effectively does), the occluded eye tends to "wander" due to the fact that the necessity to converge no longer exists. So the occlusion of the patient's left eye by the thumb of the optician must be done quickly. It is better to repeat two or three times to verify the measurement rather than to linger too long.

It is difficult for the patient to view a distant object, because the optician's head gets in the way when the two persons are directly facing one another. It is safe to say in fact that P.D.s are measured in the way they are in practice, because of the practical difficulty of following the theoretical ideal.

3.3 Rulers for semi-P.D. measurement

The previous paragraph dealing with this topic has been illustrated with the simplest form of P.D. rule, but there are other and varied rulers in existence. Probably one of the most satisfactory is the type shown in Fig. 3.10.

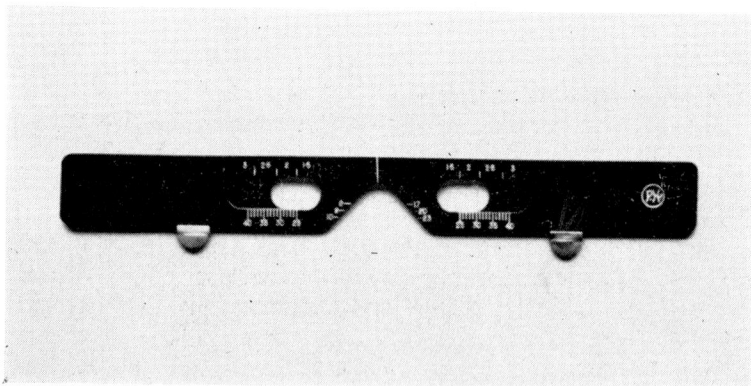

Fig. 3.10. P.D. ruler with sliding wire scale.

The thin wire mounted vertically in each aperture can be moved horizontally in each case, and the position of the wire can be read off the scale attached to each side. The advantage of this method is that it obviously measures directly in semi-P.D.s, which must be added together to give the total. The disadvantage is that parallax appears to be almost impossible to avoid, even in the most experienced hands, so that although two opticians will obtain the same total, their semi-P.D. measurements will differ. It is also once again very difficult to determine the central point of the nose, and "wobble" is very prevalent because often two hands are required.

3.4. Instruments for P.D. measurement

In addition to the rulers described in ¶3.2 and ¶3.3 for P.D. measurement, there are many other rulers and instruments ranging from simple devices to elaborate instruments capable of great accuracy and the determination of considerable ancillary data, such as the position of the frame on the face and nose, the position of the frame datum or box centre relative to the person's eyes, etc.

Some of these instruments are binocular and consist of two tubes through which the optician views in turn the two eyes of the patient. This however needs good and usable amounts of visual acuity in each eye by the optician, which may not always be available.

The two best-known elaborate instruments are the Centromatic-posimatic system by Essel of Paris, and the Zeiss Lens/Frame instrument. The reader is referred to the technical literature supplied by both companies for further information.

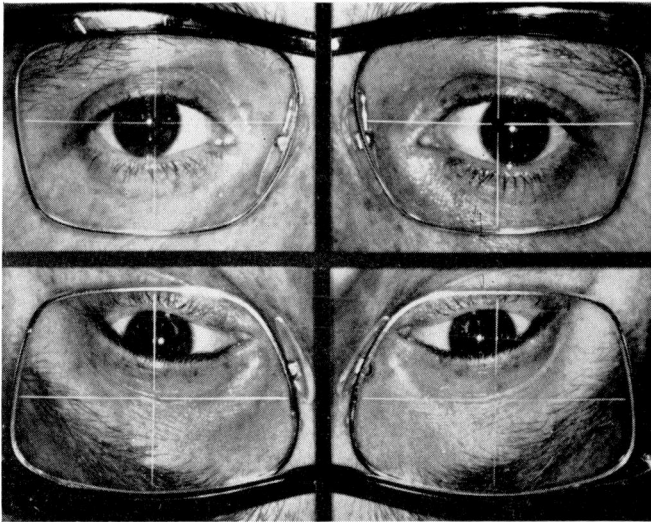

Fig. 3.11. Photograph obtained with centromatic-posimatic instrument showing frame in position, and positions of patient's eyes for distance (top) and near (bottom). (Note: Near photograph is upside down).

41

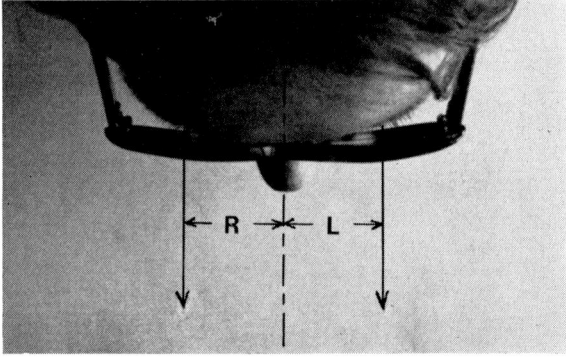
Fig. 3.12a. Frame positioned symmetrically on the face. Two semi-P.Ds. equal. 32mm. each, total 64 mm. (all measurements in the plane of the lens).

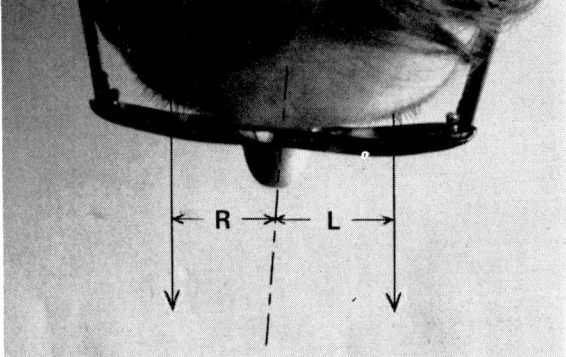
Fig. 3.12b. This case will give a reading of R. semi-P.D. 30mm. L. semi-P.D. 34mm. total 64 mm.

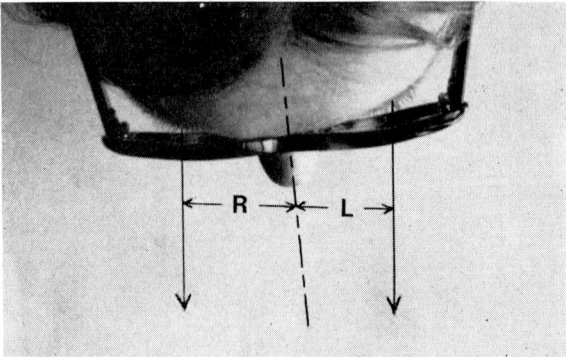
Fig. 3.12c. This will give a reading of R. semi-P.D. 34 mm. L. semi-P.D. 30 mm. total 64 mm.

3.5 Semi-P.D.

Fig. 3.12a, b and c illustrate the difficulty of determining the semi-P.D. accurately.

Fig. 3.12a shows the head situated symmetrically with regard to the antero-posterior (front to back) axis, so that the semi-P.D. measures 32 mm. for each eye.

Fig. 3.12b shows the head tilted a little to the right, so that the left semi-P.D. is greater than the right.

Fig. 3.12c shows the head tilted a little to the left, so that the right semi-P.D. is greater than the left.

When measuring a patient who requires varifocal lenses, the semi-P.D. is essential for each eye. The Centromatic-posimatic system or the Zeiss Lens/Frame instrument are both capable of determining this with great accuracy, and undoubtedly represent the ultimate yet devised for this purpose.

However, as long as great care is exercised, good results can be achieved with much more simple apparatus. This great care must be directed mainly at determining that the head of the patient and that of the optician lie in the same plane, as described earlier in this section.

Mention was made in ¶3.4 of the optician who does not possess good visual acuity in each eye, one eye perhaps being amblyopic. In this case, it is best to measure the near P.D. first (as described in ¶3.2), and the distance P.D. can then be quickly and easily calculated or determined from tables (see below ¶3.13).

In all cases, however, where any doubt exists about what the P.D. is, either due to facial asymmetry on the part of the patient, or special lenses being required, or any other circumstance, the simplest and easiest procedure is to mark up or "spot up" a frame which is either exactly what the patient requires, or very nearly so. This frame will have to be glazed with dummy plano lenses for this purpose. In fact, many frames are supplied with dummy lenses already fitted, and sometimes with the datum centres marked by means of two crossed lines either scribed in plastic or etched in glass.

43

3.6. Position of the Head

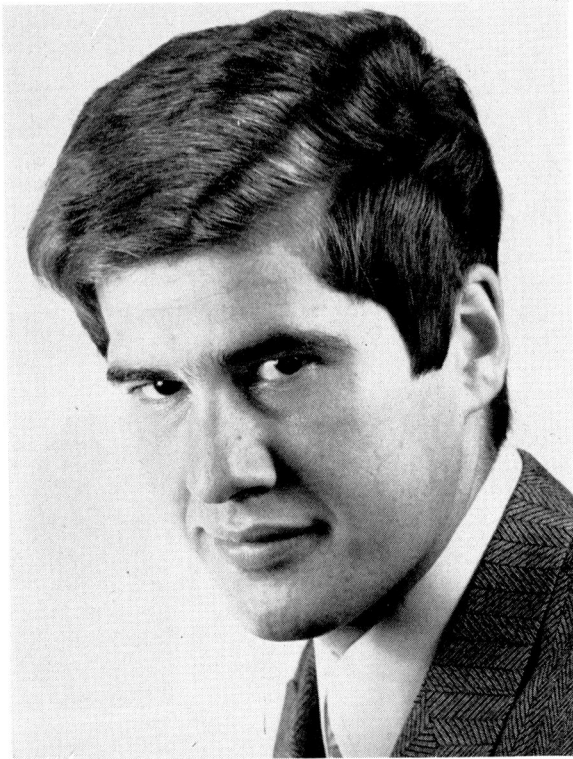

Fig. 3.13. Subject looking straight ahead with head tilted and turned sideways

Many people look straight ahead with their heads turned somewhat sideways and often tilted to one side (Fig. 3.13). This is a common feature and the optician must be on the look-out for it—even on his own part! So when measuring the P.D. care must be taken that in such a case, two different semi-P.D.s are not observed and measured. This is usually the reason for the differing semi-P.D. measurements found in the previous section.

The head of the patient must be positioned by the optician so that as nearly as he is able to judge the face of the subject is in a plane exactly parallel to his own. But if the spectacles when worn are positioned on the face which is then tilted to the right or the left with respect to the plane of fixation, it might be argued that the lenses should be mounted in the frame so that the centres correspond with the positions of the pupils in any case. This is however not usually undertaken, as will be explained later in this chapter.

44

3.7. Tolerances due to Unwanted Prismatic Effects

We will now deal with the general question of latitude to prismatic imbalance due to wrong, faulty, or deliberate misalignment of frame centres, lens centres, and the point on the lens through which the line of fixation passes. Various definitions are required (see Fig. 3.14.). D is the datum centre (already defined) O is the optical centre, i.e. the point on the lens where there is no prismatic effect. In the absence of any other information, O will be positioned $1\frac{1}{2}$ or 2 mm. above D. The horizontal distance OD, is the decentration necessary to position the optical centre of the lens in front of the pupil.

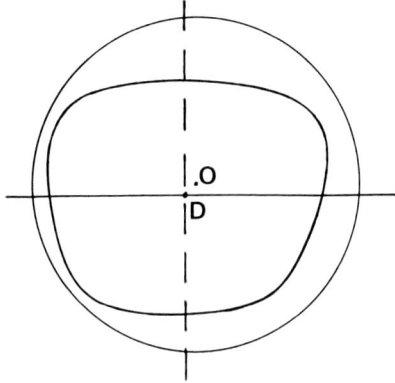

Fig. 3.14. D is the datum centre and O the optical centre of the finished lens shape, here shown imposed on the lens blank.

We are concerned at this moment with a consideration of what happens if the person looks through a point to the temporal side of one optical centre position, and to the nasal side of the other optical centre position, i.e. if effectively one lens is decentred **out** whilst the other is decentred **in.** Prentice's Rule states that P = Fc where P is the prismatic effect due to a decentration of c cm., and F the lens power.

If the patient is wearing, say, R. & L. –4.00D sph., then the prismatic effect due to turning the head to the left (but still looking forward) so that his line of fixation is say 10 mm. from the O.C. positions, then the prismatic effect will be R. 4△ base out, L. 4△ base in, and effectively the two prismatic effects cancel out.

This is always the case when the two eyes are symmetrically placed to one side or the other of the median line, and the lens power is the same. In practice, it is seldom that the two lenses are identical, but fortunately differences between the two eyes of over 3D are rare (anisometropia is the name given to the condition when there is such a marked difference). As will be seen above, 10 mm. is a somewhat extreme case, so usually much less decentration than this is involved, which therefore reduces the prismatic effect even more, and makes the problem even easier of

45

solution. Finally, even if a small extent of anisometropia is present (up to 3D), or we are involved with a fairly large amount of unwanted prismatic effects, the eye is very tolerant of prismatic effects in the horizontal plane. Due to the action of convergence, the medial and lateral rectus muscles which turn the globe on its vertical axis are much the strongest of the 6 extra-ocular muscles, and the prismatic effect which we can overcome comfortably is about $3\triangle$. For temporary periods, we can overcome $10\triangle$.

3.8. Multifocal Lenses

So far we have only dealt with single-sight lenses, except for the brief reference to varifocal lenses when dealing with other rulers for P.D. measurement. In the case of bifocals, trifocals, varifocals, etc., (usually grouped together under the heading of multifocals), other problems besides the prismatic effects of the decentred lenses arise which must receive consideration. Most notable is the fact that the eyes must look through a greater or lesser area of different power in one part of the lens from that which is present in the other part of the lens. If the semi-P.D. is wrong, then the segment or progression will be wrongly positioned, and this can lead to great difficulty. It will be seen therefore that great care in the measuring of the P.D. generally, and of the semi-P.D. under certain circumstances, is vitally important.

3.9. Vertical positioning of multifocal lenses

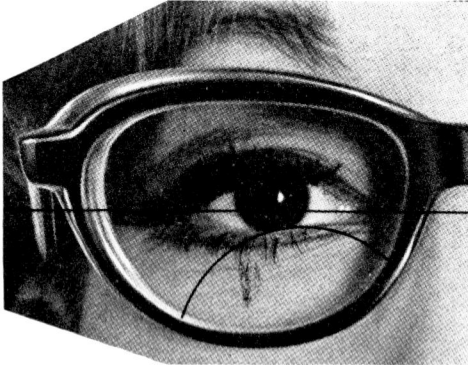

Fig. 3.15. This shows the position of a bifocal segment in normal cases.

(a) BIFOCALS. In the absence of any other consideration (an important reservation that we will return to later), and assuming a "normal" position of head and eye, it is usual to position the top of the segment 2 mm. below datum. The distance O.C. is usually positioned $1\frac{1}{2}$ mm. above datum, so that distance O.C. and segment top are separated by $3\frac{1}{2}$ mm.

46

It will be seen from Fig. 3.15 is that the distance O.C. will then be in line with the centre of the pupil, the datum line level with the lower edge of the pupil, and the segment top level with the lower edge of the iris. These positions are only approximate, as pupil sizes vary, and iris sizes are different also. However, it gives a reasonable guide to the fitting of bifocals in normal cases.

If a person holds his head up in a very upright position, the segment top must be lowered, i.e. the distance between the segment top and datum line must be increased to say 3 or 4 mm. below datum. This distance is known as the "cut".

On the other hand if a person holds his head down, or stoops, or is round-shouldered, or suffers from a physical deformity, then the cut must be decreased to say 0 or even 1 or 2 mm. above datum.

It is therefore of paramount importance to observe a person who needs bifocals with his head held in as natural a position as possible. When sitting at the fitting table to be measured for spectacles, most patients will hold their heads up unnaturally, and the dispenser must request the person to hold his head in a natural position. This is really most important, for if the bifocals are not fitted carefully, trouble will ensue. In fact if the person is measured for spectacles with his head held unnaturally high, he will drop his head when wearing the glasses, and frame and lenses will then be fitted lower than ought to be the case. The head will then probably have to be held higher than need be to enable the person to see adequately through the bifocals.

Whilst this is not good dispensing practice, it probably does not occasion the wearer a great deal of trouble in most cases. What is much worse is for the bifocals to be fitted too high in the frame, or the frame containing the bifocals to be fitted too high on the face. This causes the wearer a lot of difficulty, which may well be intolerable. Under these circumstances, the top edge of the bifocal may intrude into part of the field of view of the wearer as he looks into the distance, or slightly below it at the near distance. Above all other considerations therefore, it is imperative to position bifocals so that the pencil of light limited by the size of the pupil is uninterrupted by the segment top when looking into the near or far distance.

All the above considerations apply to what might be termed general bifocal use. Now we must look at special cases, wherein the occupation of the person requires the bifocals to be positioned differently from usual. A dentist for instance might well need a pair of spectacles with the near addition in the upper part of the frame, so that he can look upwards into his patient's mouth. This would require an "upcurve" bifocal. A librarian is sometimes in this difficulty also, being unable properly to see books on shelves above eye-level with distance glasses or conventionally fitted bifocals. An organist would require to see his music on the stand

47

in front of him, but needs a distance portion of lens also. So a bifocal fitted some 6 – 8 mm. above datum might be suggested.

It is therefore necessary to know the occupation of the person wearing bifocals, which may well influence the optician's decision or suggestion as to what type of bifocal to use, and how they should be positioned.

Fig. 3.15 illustrates a 38 mm. segment solid bifocal, and much the same conditions will apply to all round bifocal segment shapes from 22 mm. to 45 mm. In the case of the flat-top fused bifocals such as Univis or Fulvue, these may be positioned some 2 mm. lower than the round segments with no loss of effectiveness. When the eye is rotated downwards and the line of fixation passes into the bifocal segment, it passes directly into a useful area of lens and not into a restricted portion at the top. In fact, all that is being removed in the case of such flat-top bifocals is the portion of round segment that causes trouble when looking ahead or slightly downwards.

Finally, whilst discussing bifocals, it must be remarked that there are two schools of thought about the positioning of bifocal segments. One school fits the frame first, and then positions the bifocal top up or down from the standard position in order to achieve the optimum effect. The other school positions the bifocals in a standard position (except in exceptional cases), and then positions the frame up or down relative to the eyes to achieve the desired effect. Those who practise the latter argue that if the positioning of the bifocals is found to be incorrect, then the lenses may be changed to another frame of a wider D.B.L. which will cause the lenses to drop somewhat in position, or a narrower D.B.L. which will raise them. In the former case, however, if the positioning is found to be wrong it is necessary to change the lenses. In practice the good dispenser will effect a compromise between these two alternatives as the circumstances of the case dictate, bearing in mind what has been said.

(b) TRIFOCALS. Generally speaking, much that has been said about bifocals applies to trifocals also, except that the intermediate segment top is usually positioned on datum for normal cases.

(c) VARIFOCALS. The distance from the top of the progression to the start of the maximum area of reading addition varies with particular design of lens in use (usually between 8 and 12 mm.), and since the eye* has to travel downwards a considerable distance vertically on the lens before being able to see close work properly, it is usual to position the start of the progression a little above datum, between 0 – 3 mm., and to increase the reading addition usually by + 0.50D more than the amount that would be used for bifocal purposes.

*Strictly, the point of intersection of the line of fixation of the eye where this line intersects the lens.

48

3.10. Vertical Disparity in Position of the Two Eyes

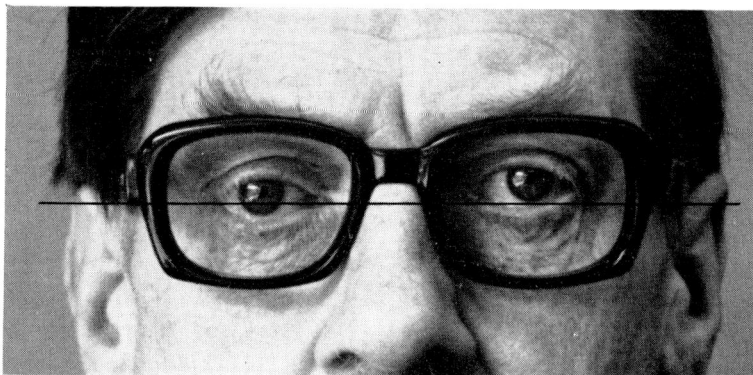

Fig. 3.16a. Frame in position on face with datum line marked. Left eye is set higher in head than right.

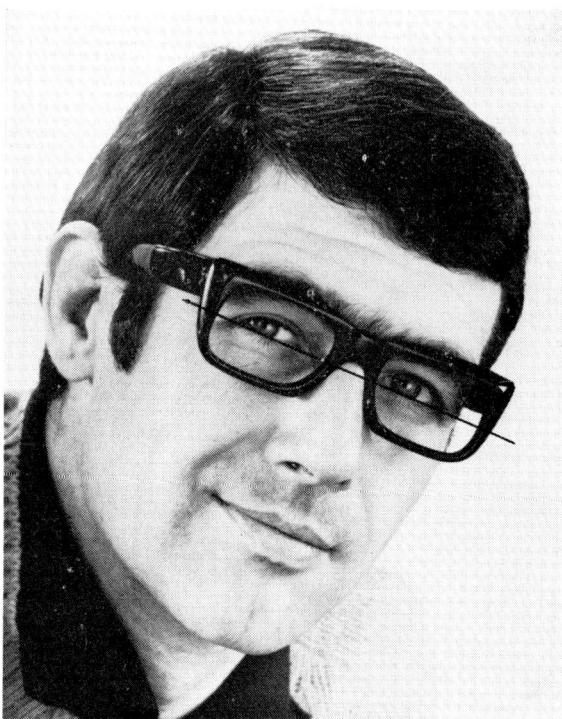

Fig. 3.16b. Frame in position on face with datum line marked. The two eyes are level with the datum line, although the head is tilted.

49

There are two cases which we must investigate here. The first (Fig. 3.16a) is where one eye (the right as illustrated) is set vertically below the other, but the face and eyebrows and bony structure are horizontally symmetrical.

The datum line of the frame made to fit comfortably and to appear correct (which will line up with the eyebrows and the contours of the face) is level with the lower edge of the right pupil and much below the left pupil.

The second case (Fig. 3.16b) is one where the left eye is below the level of the right due to the fact that the whole face is lower vertically this side than the other, including the eyebrows and bony structure. Alternatively, the head may be held tilted to one side (as illustrated).

The datum line of the frame made to fit comfortably and to appear correct (which again will line it up with the eyebrows and the contours of the face) passes just below both pupils and at the same distance below each.

The second case we can dismiss as presenting no problems. The first case definitely presents problems particularly in the event of bifocal or multifocal fitting.

Let us take the case specifically of a person having bifocals of C segment (22 mm.) positioned 2 mm. below datum in each eye. As the eyes rotate downwards, the line of fixation of the right eye will pass into the right segment whilst the left eye will still be looking through the distance portion of the left lens.

Obviously this will lead to difficulty. So care must be taken to note when measuring the P.D. to see that the two eyes are vertically aligned in the head. Any disparity should be noted, and the whole lens including the segments where necessary, decentred up or down accordingly. In the case of our example, Fig. 3.16a, the right lens would need bodily decentration downwards.

3.11. Vertical Position of Lenses in Frames

To sum up: it is normal practice to position the distance optical centre $1\frac{1}{2}$ – 2 mm. above the datum centre in the absence of any contrary information (confirm with your Prescription House). The datum centre should be positioned in normal cases in line with the lower edge of the pupil, so that the optical centre coincides with the pupil centre. The lens will be glazed eccentrically as required in order to introduce any decentration necessary to enable this to be achieved.

Bifocals should be positioned so that the segment top is 2 mm. below the datum line in normal cases. Flat-top bifocals may be positioned lower so as to provide a more uninterrupted distance vision. However, where the person has a different stance from normal, or where the visual requirements are such as to require the greater emphasis to be given to near vision rather than to distance vision, due allowance must be made.

Varifocal lenses are usually positioned with the start of the progression on or a little above datum (treat every case as an individual one), and determine as carefully as possible the relative importance to be attached to distance/near visual requirements, remembering that the maximum area of reading addition is not reached until 8 – 12 mm. below the distance O.C. (depending upon the type of varifocal).

3.12. Near Vision Lenses

Presbyopia is that condition of the eye which starts in the middle years of life (about 45 years of age) and progresses until about 65 years of age. Due to difficulty in focusing rays of light on to the macula (caused by sclerosing of the lens and other associated factors), a convex powered supplementary lens is required in front of the eye to make good the deficiency. If a distance correction is worn, then a reading "addition" is required to the distance Rx.

The eyes are normally rotated downwards when reading, so that the line of fixation passes through the lenses at a point some 8 – 12 mm. below the datum line (This is the N.V.P., the near visual point). It might be argued that logically as well as inward decentration to allow for convergence, a downward decentration to allow for the depression of the eyes in reading, should be necessary. However a little thought will show that the same sort of condition arises here as in the case discussed under the heading of "tolerance due to unwanted prismatic effects", ¶3.7. Usually both lenses are of much the same power, so a prismatic effect at the N.V.P. of approximately the same amount vertically will be introduced if no vertical decentration is carried out. The imbalance between the two eyes is therefore normally either nil or negligible. There is thus no useful purpose served by decentring downwards lenses required for reading only—unless there is a considerable amount of anisometropia present. Even in this case, with no downward decentration given, the spectacle wearer will lower his head to bring the visual axes into coincidence with the optical centres to avoid discomfort caused by unwanted prismatic effects. Downward decentration will never be given therefore except in very exceptional circumstances.

3.13. Relation between Distance P.D. and Near P.D.

The following table gives the relationship between the distance P.D. and the near P.D. for varying P.Ds. and distances.

INTER–PUPILLARY DISTANCES

DISTANCE	MUSIC (INTERMEDIATE)		READING OR WRITING	
6 metres and infinity	900 mm. (violin)	500 mm. (piano)	400 mm. (desk)	300 mm. (book)
51	50	49	48	47
53	51	50	49	48
54	52	51	50	49
55	53	52	51	50
56	54	53	52	51
57	55	54	53	52
58	56	55	53.5	52.5
59	57	56	54	53
60	58	57	55	54
61	59	58	56	55
62	60	59	57	56
63	61	59.5	58	57
64	62	60.5	59	58
65	63	61	60	59
66	64	62	61	60
67	65	63	62	61
68	66	64	63	62
69	67	65	64	63
70	68	66	65	64
71	69	67	66	65
72	70	68	67	66
73	71	69	68	67
74	72	70	69	68
75	73	71	69.5	68.5
76	74	72	70	69

CHAPTER IV

FRAME MEASUREMENTS

4.1. Frame Styles and Types

Whilst frames are, and indeed have to be, specified in terms of eyesize, datum centre distance (dat. C.D.), distance between lenses (D.B.L.), bridge type and measurement, position of joint, length of side, etc., etc., it is equally if not more important to specify them in terms of style. This to a large extent is not within the control of the optician, who must specify a frame style usually by the name given by the manufacturer of that particular frame. The name automatically identifies the frame, and many if not all of the features associated with it, such as thickness of material, colours, whether monotone or two-tone (if plastics), type of side, etc. Consequently familiarity with frame styles is probably one of the major requirements of a good dispenser, and only long experience can supply this.

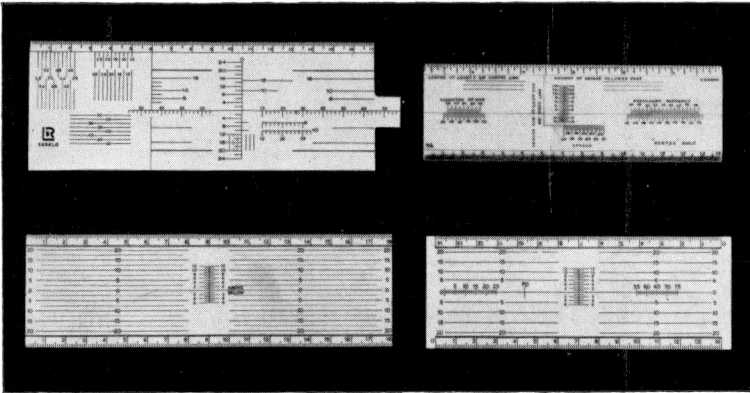

Fig. 4.1. Various frame rulers.

53

4.2. Frame Rulers

There are many and varied rulers in existence. Four different patterns have been illustrated in Fig. 4.1, and one in particular has been selected, Fig. 4.2a, to demonstrate the technique of frame measuring to be described in the following paragraphs.

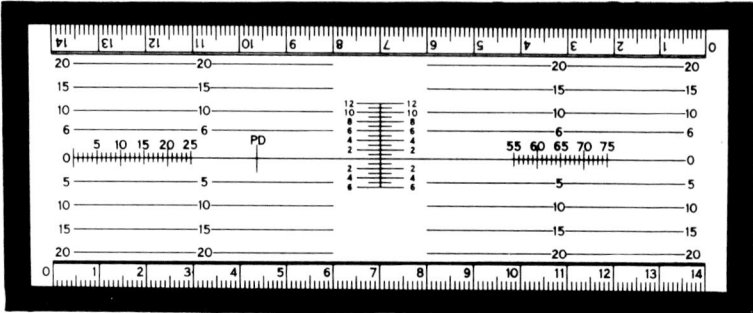

Fig. 4.2a. Frame ruler used in following text.

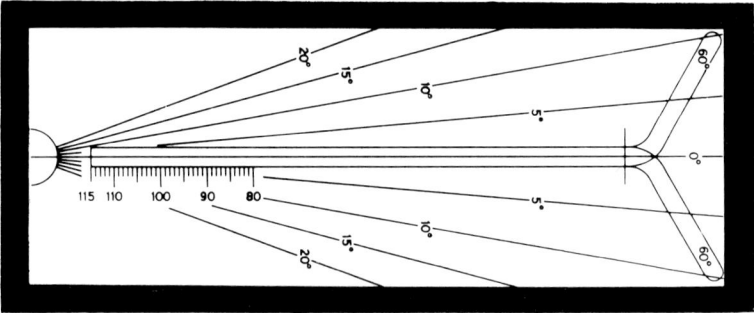

Fig. 4.2b. Reverse side of Fig. 4.2a.

This rule has a millimetre scale along one edge. An upside down scale is marked along the top edge, so that when turned over it still measures from left to right.

The datum line is ruled along the middle, and equidistant from this line are others drawn at 5, 10, 15 and 20 mm. intervals. The exception to this is the line drawn 6 mm. above the datum line on the left hand side.

In order to measure a spectacle frame, it is necessary to know where the datum line lies. The datum line of the ruler, and the equidistant lines

54

drawn on it, are to enable this to be done, as will be described in the next para. 4.3. The line drawn 6 mm. above the datum line is to enable the spread of regular bridges to be determined (see ¶4.4. & ¶4.5).

In the centre of the ruler, vertically above and below the datum line, are a series of small horizontal lines at 1 mm. intervals, and marked more prominently every 2 mm., with numbers 2, 4, 6, 8, 10 & 12 above, and 2, 4 & 6 below. These are for bridge heights to be determined. (see ¶4.4. & ¶4.5).

To the left of the bridge height scale, is a small vertical line marked **P.D.** From this line to the right is the measurement of frame P.D. or frame dat. C.D. (datum centre distance). (see ¶4.4). Frames of dat. C.D. below 55 mm. or above 75 mm. are almost non-existent, so only measurements within these limits have been indicated.

To the left of the datum line is a series of marks, 5, 10, 15, 20 & 25 used for determining regular bridge spread measurements at 6 mm. below the long horizontal line parallel to the datum line previously referred to. The position of the zero might with advantage be inserted in this scale.

On the reverse side of the ruler, Fig. 4.2b, is a further set of lines to determine the joint angle, length of side, etc. This is described in ¶4.10 et seq, and the illustrations should be clear without the necessity for further description here.

4.3. Frame Measurements (All measurements in millimetres)

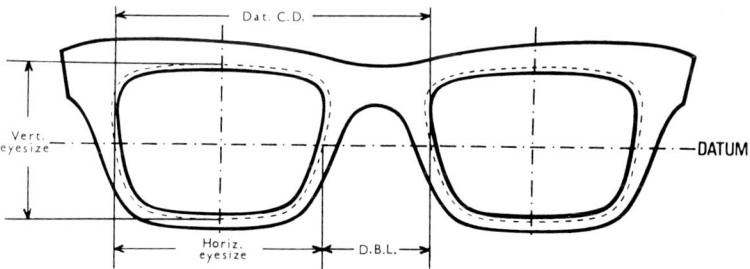

Fig. 4.3. Frame front showing relationship between dat. C.D., D.B.L. and eyesize.

The three most important measurements **always** are:-

    (a) eyesize (horizontal)
    (b) datum centre distance (dat. C.D.)   } (a) + (c) = (b)
    (c) distance between lenses (D.B.L.)

The connections between these three measurements may be seen from Fig. 4.3 above. The dat. C.D. (variously termed the Frame P.D., or Frame Centre (F.C.) distance) is measured in the same way as the P.D. of a person, i.e. from one inside rim on datum, to the corresponding point on the opposite rim. It should be noted that the eyesize is the size of the glazed lens which in the case of V-edged lenses, is from the bottom of the groove on one side of the datum line, to the bottom of the groove on the other side. The vertical lens measurement through the datum centre should also be given if required. It is imperative in the case of a hand-made special frame, or where there is any possibility of doubt.

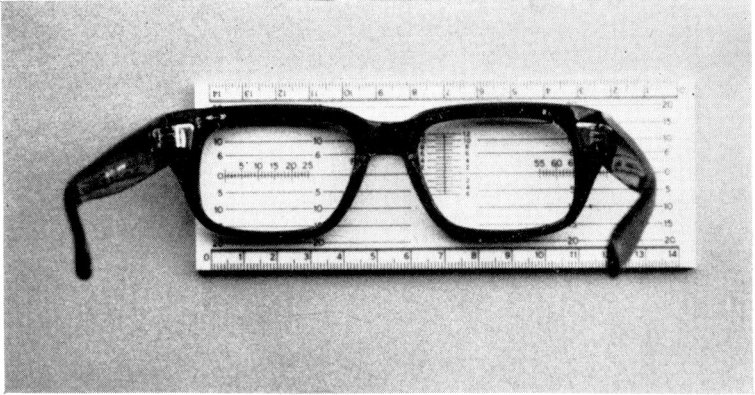

Fig. 4.4a. Frame placed on ruler.

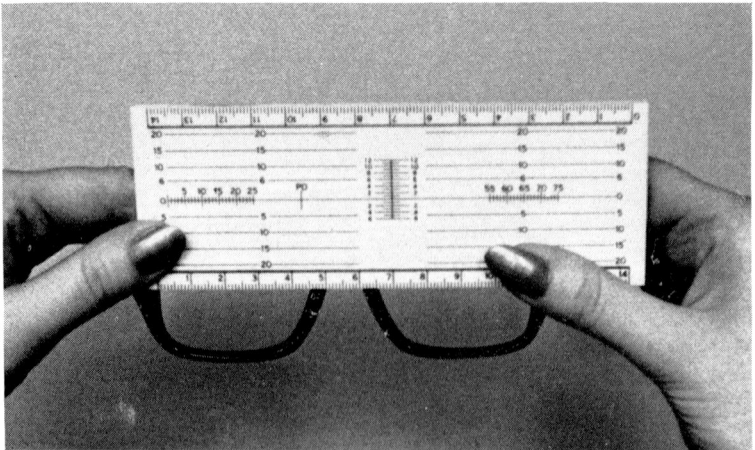

Fig. 4.4b. Ruler placed against frame.

In order to undertake these measurements, one of two methods may be adopted.

(a) First method. Frame placed on ruler. (Fig. 4.4a). There are a number of horizontal lines on the ruler, and the frame should be positioned so that **when viewed directly from above,** i.e. so that there is no parallax, the datum line is positioned equidistantly from the inside of the top and bottom rims. The dat. C.D. may then be determined from the appropriate markings on the ruler, being from the nasal side of the left lens to the temporal side of the right lens.

(b) Second method. Ruler placed against frame. (Fig. 4.4b). With a reasonable amount of practice, the position of the datum line may be gauged sufficiently accurately by eye, so that the ruler may be placed along the datum line of the frame, and the eyesize and dat. C.D. read off from the edge scale of the ruler.

As remarked before, in spite of the standards which have been laid down, there is considerable variation between different manufacturers in the measurements given to frames, and a frame ostensibly 44 eyesize (horizontal) $\times$ 64 dat. C.D. (20 D.B.L.), may be found to be 43, 44 or 45 on datum. Most manufacturers of mass produced frames stamp the eyesize and dat. C.D. or D.B.L. on the inside of the front, or attach small self-adhesive labels to the inside of the side. When specifying a frame measurement, it is advisable to adhere to the measurements given by the manufacturer to that frame.

Apart from eyesize and dat. C.D. or D.B.L., which are common to all frame styles and types, the further measurements required will depend on the material of the frame, type of bridge, and other factors discussed below.

As has been pointed out already, there many other rulers in existence besides those illustrated in Fig. 4.1. or used in Figs. 4.2a and 4.2b. The measurements of dat. C.D., D.B.L. and eyesize however are basic to all frames, and the methods described above using the particular rules concerned, may be applied to all other rulers.

4.4. Plastics frames (and tortoiseshell frames)

There are two main patterns, pad bridge frames and regular bridge frames.

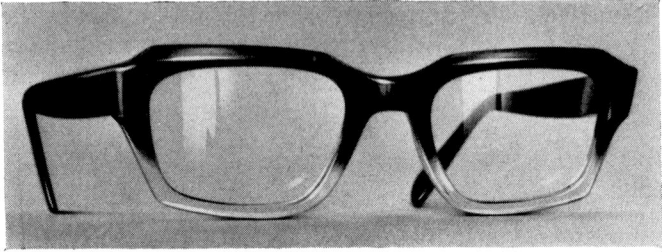

Fig. 4.5a. Pad bridge plastics frame, arch pad.

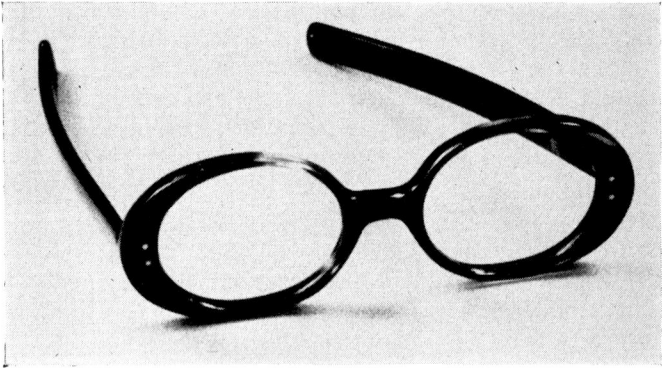

Fig. 4.5b. Regular bridge plastics frame.

(a) Pad bridge plastics frame (front measurements).

		B.S. Ref. No.
(i)	Eyesize (horizontal and vertical)	(4103)
(ii)	Dat. C.D. (datum centre distance)	(4106)
(iii)	D.B.L. (distance between lenses)	(4104)
(iv)	D.B.R. (distance between rims) on datum	(6101)
(v)	D.B.R. at specified distances below datum	(6101)
(vi)	Projection of bridge (from back plane of front)	(4109)

58

		B.S. Ref. No.
(vii)	Height of lower edge of bridge centre above datum	(4108)
(viii)	Height of tops of pads above datum	(6301)
(ix)	Splay of pads	(6106)
(x)	Length of pads (overall length top to bottom)	—
(xi)	Type of pads	—
(xii)	Width of pads	(6303)
(xiii)	Frontal angle of pad	(6105)

The above measurements are common to the two main types of pad bridge frames, arch pad and keyhole pad. If a keyhole pad is to be specified, a further measurement is required:-

		B.S. Ref. No.
(xiv)	Distance between pad tops above datum	(6302)
	e.g. 14 @ 4 means 14 mm. apart at 4 mm. above datum.	

(v) to (xiv) are relatively not so important, and often may be omitted since they are invariably standard to any particular type of frame. Thus they must be accepted if this type of frame is required. However if special measurements are necessary, they may be specified as required.

Measurements above datum are + whilst those below are —, so for example (viii) may have a minus measurement.

(xiii) is an important measurement since this will usually determine the "snugness" of the fit of the frame down the bearing surface of the side of the nose. If the angle is too steep, the frame will rest on the lower edge of the pads and not at the top. If too shallow, the frame will rest on the upper edge of the pads and not on the lower. Consequently a measurement of the frontal angle of pad will often determine immediately whether a frame may be accepted or rejected as being capable of providing a comfortable fit. (see also ¶5.4).

(b) Regular (or ordinary) bridge plastics frame (front measurements).

		B.S. Ref. No.
(i)	Eyesize (horizontal and vertical)	(4103)
(ii)	Dat. C.D. (datum centre distance)	(4106)
(iii)	D.B.L. (distance between lenses)	(4104)
(iv)	Height of bridge above datum	(4108)
(v)	Projection of bridge (from back plane of front)	(4109)
(vi)	Base and depth of bridge (measured below crest) (often called spread measurement)	(5201)
(vii)	Apical radius	(5202)
(viii)	Angle of crest	(4110)

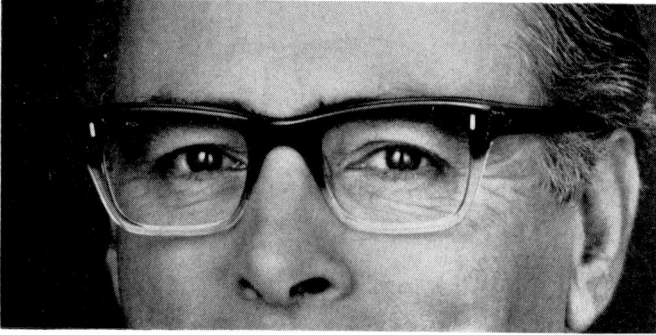

Fig. 4.6a. Pad bridge fitting.

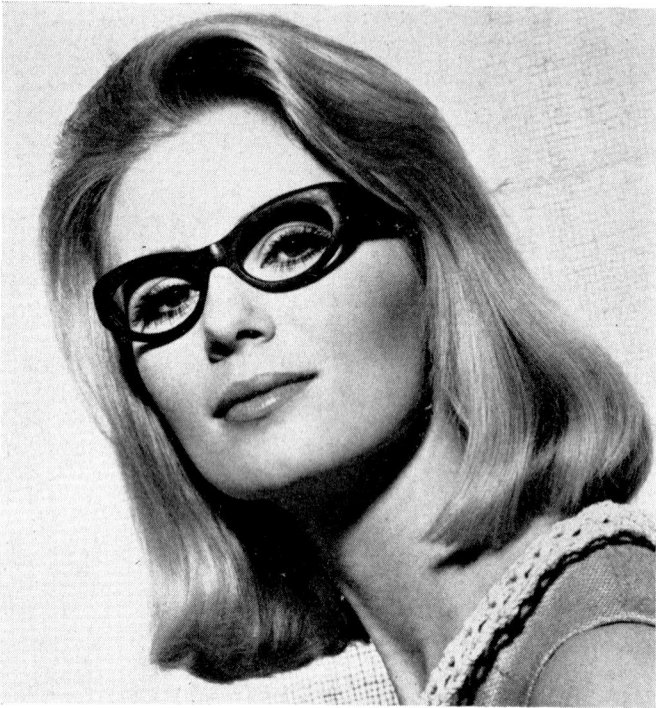

Fig. 4.6b. Pad bridge frame with low bridge height, giving fitting similar to regular bridge.

4.5 Note about difference between pad bridge and regular bridge fitting.

The main difference between a pad bridge fitting and a regular bridge fitting concerns the bearing surface of the frame and its position on the nose of the person wearing it.

A pad bridge fitting rests on the two pads on each side of the nose. The frontal angle should be such that the whole of the bearing surface of the pads rests on the side of the nose from top to bottom (or as nearly as possible). The D.B.L. should be such that the datum line of the frame is brought into the required position relative to the eyes. If the D.B.L. is too wide, the frame will drop; if too narrow, the frame will be too high.

A regular bridge fitting rests all round the bridge of the person's nose, both round the top of the bridge and down each side. It will be determined largely by the shape of the nose. A measurement of 16 @ 6 for example tells us that the space inside and under the bridge is to be 16 mm. wide at 6 mm. below the crest of the bridge. This is known as the base and depth of the bridge or the spread measurement. This will then fit around the shape of the patient's nose. Many opticians prefer to give base or spread measurements at 10 mm. and 15 mm. below crest, as this provides better control of the shape of the bridge of the frame.

Note the essential difference therefore. A pad bridge frame requires a D.B.L. measured with respect to datum. A regular bridge fitting requires a spread measured below the crest.

Many examples of regular bridge fittings have been illustrated throughout the book (Figs. 2.4 a, b & c, and Figs. 5.3 a, b & c).

However, particularly if a pad bridge frame is made with a fairly low bridge, e.g. 4 – 6 mm. above datum, it is possible with careful selection to fit a pad bridge snugly around the nose so that it achieves the same sort of fitting that a regular bridge is designed to provide. Such a fitting has been shown in Fig. 4.6b.

The same sort of circumstance will also arise in a pad frame with the more normal bridge height of 10 – 12 mm. above datum, if the person has a high bridge. Fig. 4.6a in fact is again an almost perfect example of a regular bridge fitting achieved with a pad bridge because the person has a high and well-defined bridge around which the frame fits very well.

4.6. Inset bridge for regular bridge fitting, plastics frames

Sometimes it is found that even a 0 projection (i.e. a flush bridge) will allow a frame to rest on the cheeks, or the lashes to touch the lenses, etc. In this case, it is necessary to build the bridge up into what is known as an inset bridge.

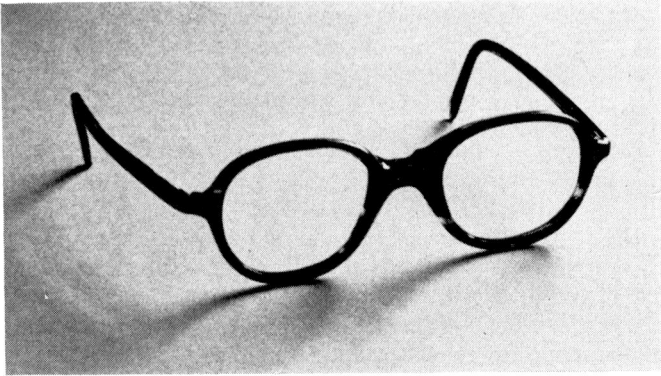

Fig. 4.7a. Inset bridge frame, regular bridge fitting, front view.

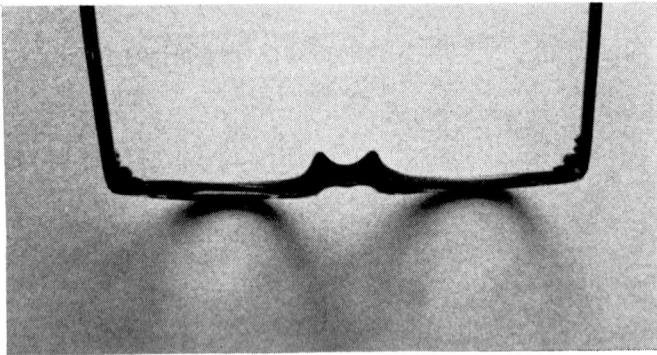

Fig. 4.7b. Inset bridge frame, regular bridge fitting, plan view.

The bridge height and spread may be given as before. The projection is the distance (in the vertical plane) from the centre of the bridge to the back plane of the front. In Fig. 4.7, the inset projection is —3. The full bridge measurements are 2 × —3, 14 @ 6. It will usually be found that a person who requires an inset bridge has no well-defined bridge to the nose.

62

4.7. Plastics frames. half-eye patterns

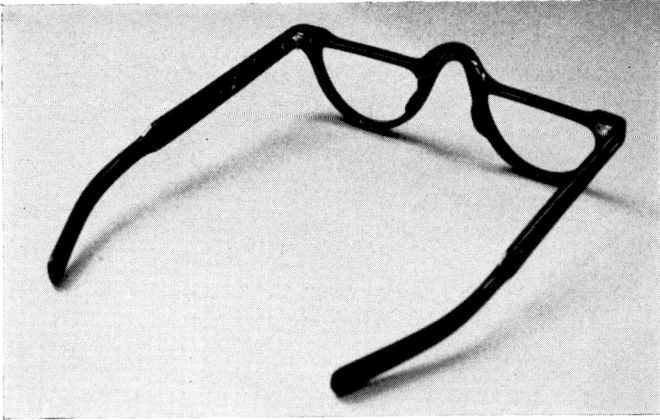

Fig. 4.8a. Plastics half-eye pad frame.

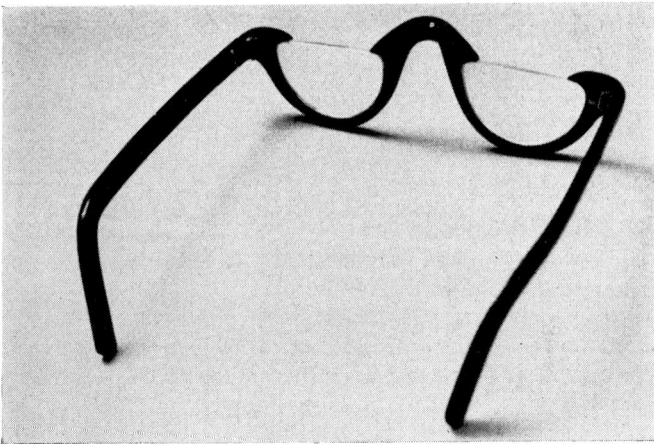

Fig. 4.8b. Plastics half-eye regular bridge supra frame.

Datum measurements do not apply to this type of frame, the style of which is not suitable. Measurements are made with respect to box sizes, i.e. 40 × 20 would indicate a lens size of 40 mm. maximum horizontal width and 20 mm. maximum depth.

As there is no datum line, bridge heights must be measured relative to some other fixed line, so the top of the lens is usually taken as the axis of reference. Due to variation in size and position of joint, it is not usually advisable to consider the centre line of joint as the horizontal axis, although this is sometimes used. Pad bridge measurements or regular bridge measurements are then made as before.

4.8. Metal Frames

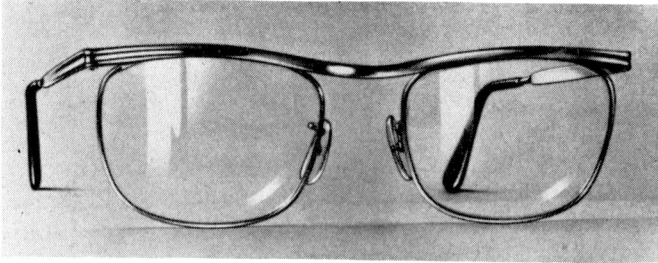

Fig. 4.9a. Pad bridge metal frame.

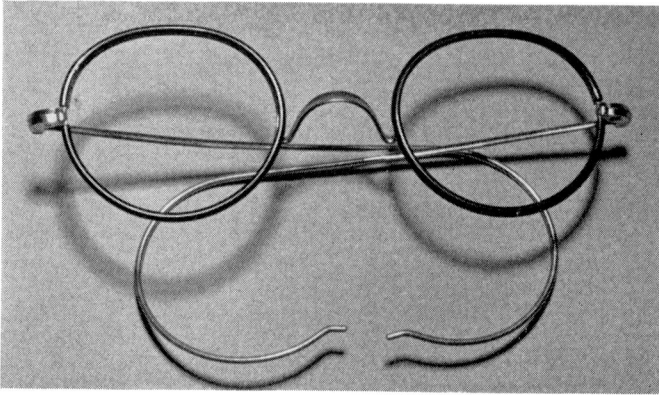

Fig. 4.9b. Regular bridge metal frame.

(a) Pad bridge metal frame. There is little or no control over position, size, etc. of the pads, which are almost invariably standard to the type of frame required. (There are one or two minor exceptions to this rule).
(b) Regular bridge metal frame: usually known as a W bridge.

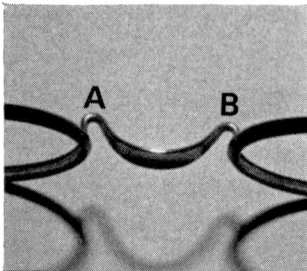

Fig. 4.10. Metal W bridge.

Measurements required:-	B.S. Ref. No.
(i) Eyesize	(4103)
(ii) Dat C.D.	(4106)
(iii) Bridge height above datum	(4108)
(iv) Bridge proj. from back plane of front	(4109)
(v) Depth of bridge	(5102)
(vi) Distance apart of A and B	(5101)
(vii) Angle of crest	(4110)
(viii) Apical radius	(5103)

Metal frames are also available in half-eye patterns.

4.9. Supra Frames

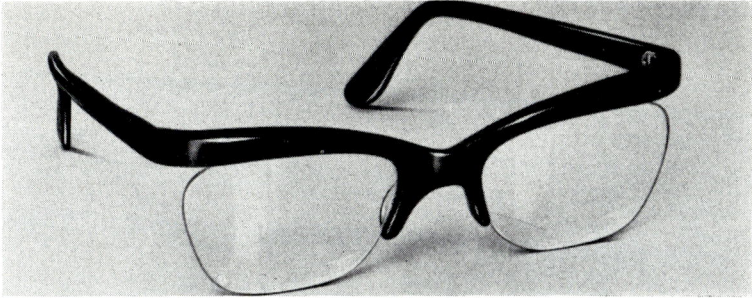

Fig. 4.11a. Supra plastics frame, pad bridge.

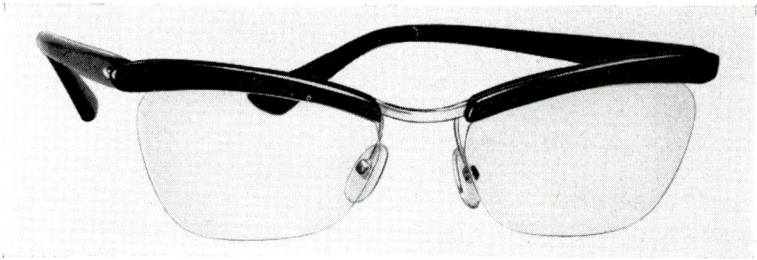

Fig. 4.11b. Supra combination "Polymil" pad frame.

As before, there are two types of bridge, regular bridge and pad bridge. Fig. 4.11a illustrates a pad bridge frame.

Since the introduction of the first supra pattern frame shortly after 1945, this style has achieved wide-scale popularity. Fig. 4.11b illustrates one of the more sophisticated derivatives, under the name of Polymil, wherein a plastics lens is bonded to a plastics insert which is fastened into the brow-bar of the frame concerned. There are many other types and patterns based upon the same idea of a rimless lower portion to the lens.

4.10. Joints and Joint Angle

The joint position may vary from central to high. There is not a great deal of variation in most frames of the same style. Consequently specification of the frame style will automatically place the joint in the position it has to occupy.

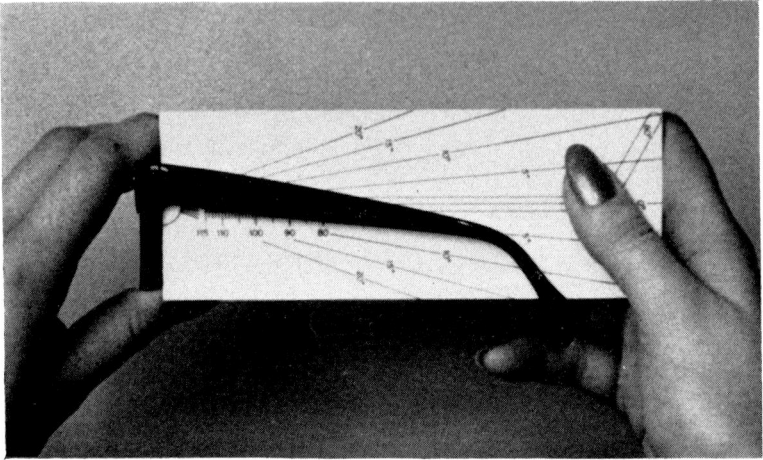

Fig. 4.12 Measurement of joint angle.

Fig. 4.12 shows the frame placed in position on the ruler to measure the joint angle.

It will be observed that the joint angle is measured along the lower edge of the side from the bottom of the dowel point (or bottom of the screw) to the normal to the front. It is shown as 7° in Fig. 4.12.

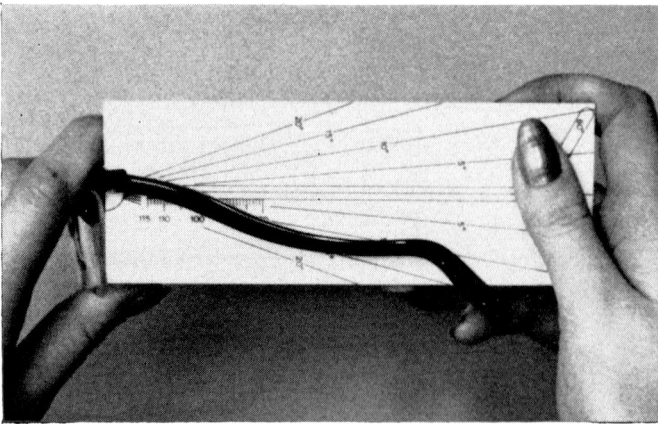

Fig. 4.13. Measurement of joint angle for sinuous sides.

66

Fig. 4.13 shows a sinuous side frame placed in position on the ruler. In this type of frame, the joint angle is the angle formed at the dowel point with the normal to the front, and the line from the dowel point to the bottom of the side at bend. It is shown as 12° in Fig. 4.13.

4.11. Sides

The overall length of side is the total of two measurements:-
(a) length from dowel point to bend (called length to bend).
(b) length from bend to finish (called length of drop).
Sometimes in the case of straight sides, or many Continental frames, an overall length only is specified.

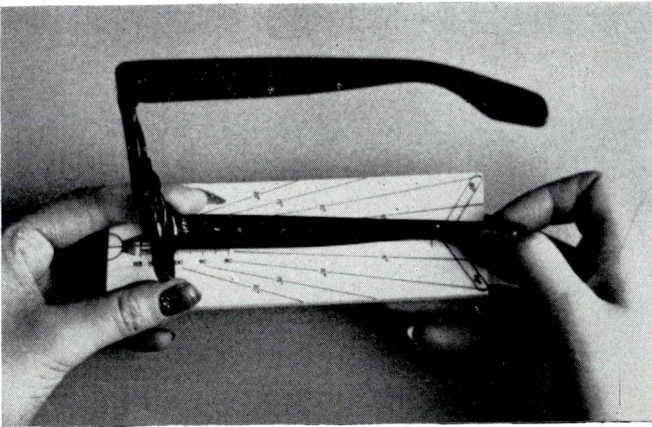

Fig. 4.14. Measurement of length of side.

Some sides are very wide at the joint, and do not have a very pronounced bend, so the position of the bend is difficult to determine with accuracy. The ruler illustrated shows how this may be ascertained. The side is placed on the rule with the **beginning** of the bend at the position of the small vertical mark as shown. The length of side is measured back to the dowel point. This conforms to the stipulation that the length of side from dowel point to ear point shall be the required measurement. It is 100 mm. to bend in Fig. 4.14.

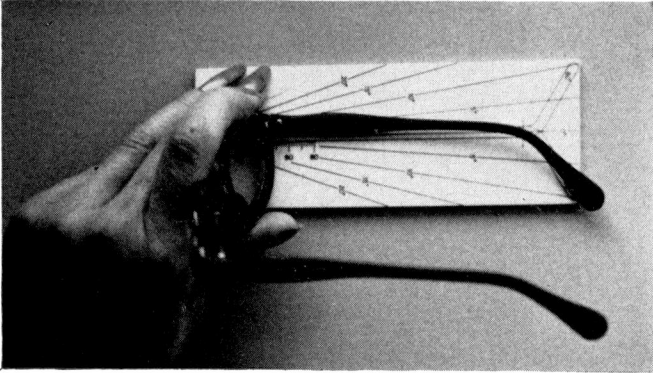

Fig. 4.15. Measurement of angle of drop.

The angle of drop is the angle as shown in Fig. 4.15, between the vertica'
and the underneath of the side at the ear point, being approximately
40° as shown. As long as the overall length of side is correct the length
of drop and angle of drop may be achieved by adjustment when finally
fitted on the client.

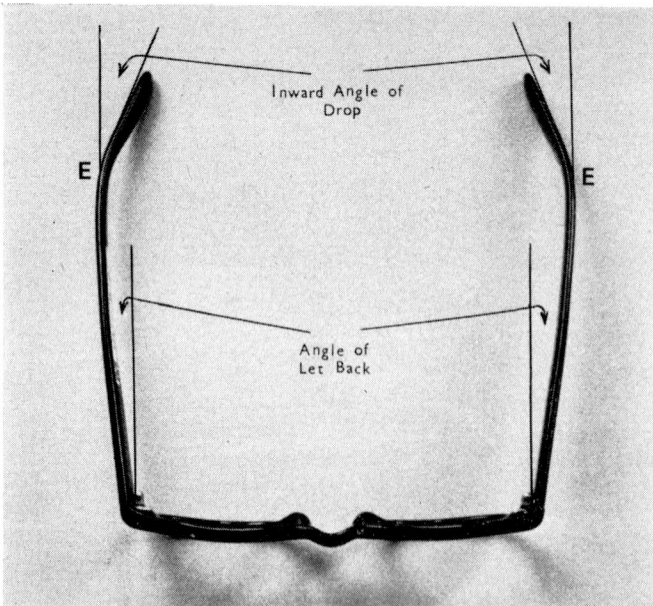

Fig. 4.16. Frame with sides open to show angle of let back of sides
and inward angle of drop.

The angle of let back of the sides is shown in Fig. 4.16, being R.6°, L.8°.

The inward angle of drop is also illustrated in Fig. 4.16, being 22° each side. E E are the ear points.

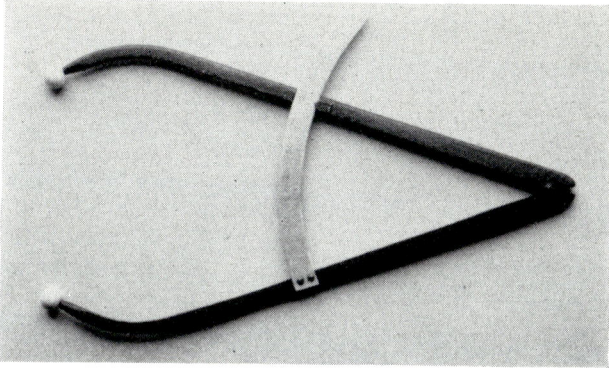

Fig. 4.17. Temple width measure.

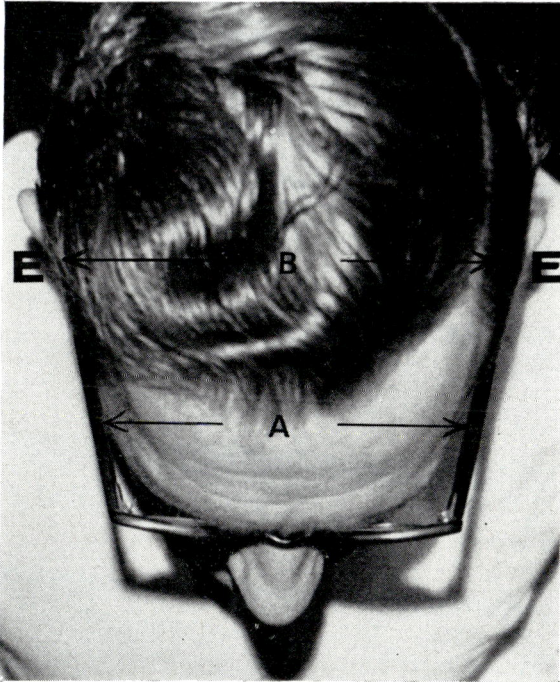

Fig. 4.18. Temple widths at A and B.

69

The distance A in Fig. 4.18 is usually known as the temple width and the distance B as the head width. Various distances from the plane of the front may be used or understood for T.W. measurements. However it should be noted that whereas in Fig. 4.18, the distance of 25 mm. from the back plane of the front will give a fixed position of A from the front, the distance B of the ear points E E from the front will vary with different individuals.

4.12. Other Measurements

In spite of the detailed nature of the measurements listed in the previous paragraphs 4.2 to 4.11, there are occasions when other measurements are required. These may refer to thickness of the material of the front, e.g. 3 or $3\frac{1}{2}$ mm. material is usually used for ordinary weight frames, and this may be required to be, say, 5 mm. Sides may be 10 mm. wide at the joints and may be required to be 15 mm. wide. The permutations are infinite. In such cases, as long as the requirements are quite specific and a sample, or if in doubt a precise sketch of what is required, is enclosed with the order, the frame maker will be able to make the frame.

CHAPTER V

FRAME FITTING

5.1. Frame details necessary for satisfactory fitting.

The determination of frame measurements necessary for satisfactory fitting is a combination of cosmetic features, i.e. how a frame "looks", thickness of material, colour of material (i.e. a light material or a metal or a supra frame may be supplied in a larger size than a dark monotone frame), shape of lens, purpose for which required, prescription to be filled, and many other features. It is quite impossible therefore to lay down exact rules for the guidance of dispensers, as each case will vary insofar as these requirements will need to receive attention. The next chapter (Chapter 6) will attempt to give such guidance, but only in broad outline.

Certain matters may however be dealt with now, but it is essential to point out that it is not intended to infer that these are the only points which should receive consideration. It is that these are perhaps capable of fairly precise quantitative measurements, and so are definitive. Other points are a matter of opinion, both of optician and of patient, and a considerable amount of give and take, freedom of choice and discussion must ensue before a decision is to be reached.

Satisfactory frame fitting can only be achieved with a reasonable selection and assortment of sample frames of different styles, shapes, sizes, materials and so on. The patient has to wear the finished article, and this fact weighs very heavily in the decision which has to be taken. Fashion and appearance are of paramount importance.

Assuming that a decision has been reached as to the style, size, colour, etc., the measurements needed must then be determined. A suggested procedure is now indicated.

5.2. Eyesize.

The frame style must obviously have been chosen at this stage, and the style will usually limit the measurements necessary. For example, if a pad bridge library frame is required, then it is useless measur-

71

ing for bridge height, projection, spread below crest, and so on. N.B. "Library" is the term applied to heavy weight plastics or tortoiseshell frames, usually with wide sides.

The first thing to do, therefore, having decided upon the frame style, is to look at the frame on the person's face to see if the size looks correct. This is a matter of opinion. Two opticians may differ in their assessment of this essential point. Two patients will almost certainly differ in their ideas. One of the most important points by which it is possible to be guided is to observe the size of any previous frame which has been worn. From the point of appearance, it may not matter if the final frame dispensed is larger than the original, but it will seldom be accepted by the wearer if it is smaller.

For many years during the 1950 – 1970 period, the tendency was for frame sizes gradually to become larger and larger. Eventually sizes have been reached where there is considerable difficulty in fitting lenses which will provide the correct optical effects. This point will not be elaborated here, but will be dealt with at greater length in Chapter 7.

A reasonable lens size is chosen usually with the active participation of the subject who will generally have his own ideas—which may not necessarily be those of the optician! When in doubt, always provide the larger eyesize, unless considerations such as weight or decentration become important.

5.3. Colour.

The decision as to the colour or colours is particularly important in the case of ladies. It has been found as a general rule that it is best usually to leave this to the patient, with perhaps merely helpful comments and observations from the optician. Most frames are available in a range of colours, and many people will want to see all the colours available before they make up their minds. Even then, they may decide they want something else, but it is not advisable to make specially any frames or colours which cannot be shown to the person.

From experience we know that such people are the difficult ones (perhaps not intentionally, and they may be most charming with it). Nevertheless, having gone to the trouble and expense of making such a frame, to find that it is not what is wanted anyway is most frustrating. So the firm advice is to adhere rigidly to the colours and sizes in which standard frames are made, and not try to be too helpful!

The point of keeping to standard colours and sizes is that if a person does not like the finished frame for any reason, it can then be fairly easily changed for another frame of a different colour in the same size, whilst the original frame is put into stock for display purposes or for subsequent further use. This cannot easily be done with spectacles made to individual requirements.

There is one general exception to this rule, and that concerns the person whose facial measurements are such that the standard sizes of frames will not fit or look correct. In this sort of condition, the optician has no option but to make a frame specially.

5.4. Bridge fittings

(a) Pad Bridge. The next point to receive consideration is the fit of the frame on the bridge of the nose. If the frame is too high, a pad bridge frame will need to be wider, and conversely if the frame is too low, the bridge will need to be narrower.

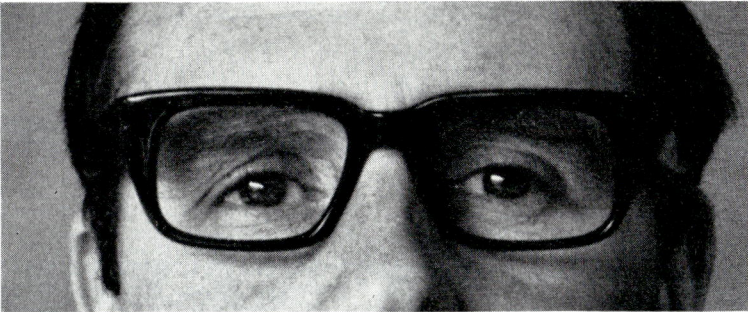

Fig. 5.1a. Frame too high, pad bridge too narrow.

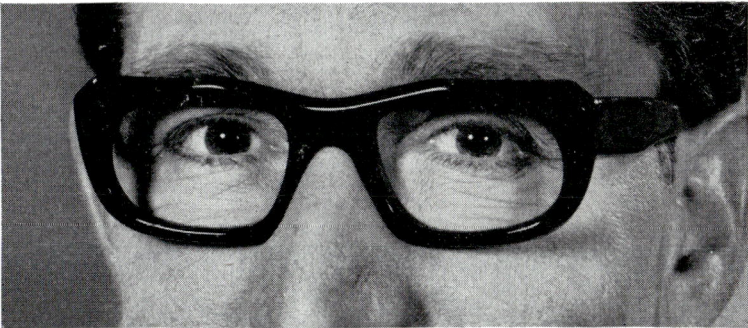

Fig. 5.1b. Frame too low, pad bridge too wide.

In Fig. 5.1a is illustrated a frame which needs to be positioned lower down by fitting a wider bridge. In Fig. 5.1b the frame needs to be positioned higher by fitting a narrower bridge. Pad bridge fittings are usually desig-

73

nated by D.B.L. measurements. 20, 22, 24 D.B.L. are the usual sizes, although in some popular frames, the range may be 18, 20, 22, 24, 26. However, many frames are only made in a limited range, or even a single D.B.L. Added to the eyesize, this gives the dat. C.D. (datum centre distance).

If special measurements are required, the D.B.L. should be quoted, together with the D.B.R. on datum, and at specified distances below datum.

Sometimes it is found that the spread of the bridge is too broad or too narrow, i.e. the frontal angle of the pad bridge is too great or too little. In a broad spread, Fig. 5.2a, the frame may rest correctly on the bridge on datum, but be too wide say at 10 mm. below datum. This is very clearly shown in the illustration where the gap between the side of the bridge of the frame and the nose is obviously visible towards the lower extremities of the pads.

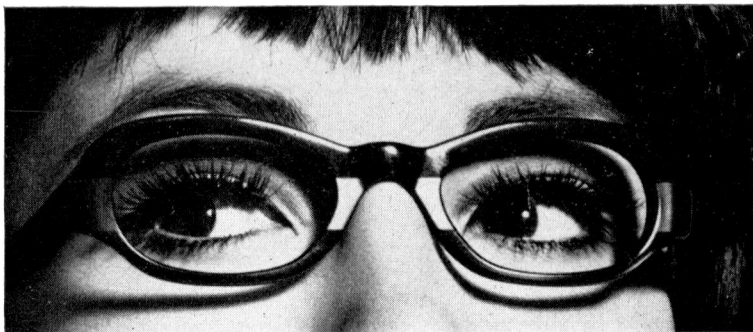

Fig. 5.2a. Frame correct height, but spread of pad bridge too broad.

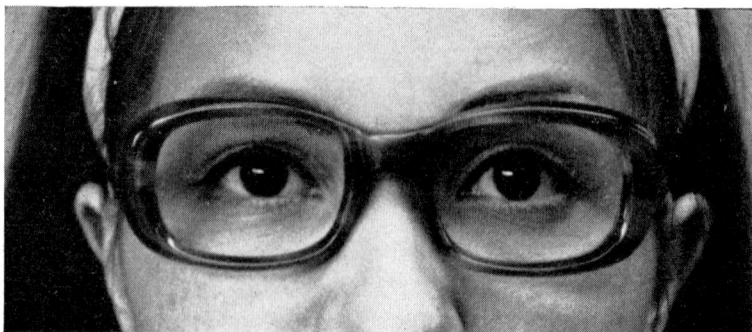

Fig. 5.2b. Frame correct height, but spread of pad bridge too narrow.

A narrower D.B.L. will result in the frame resting on a lower part of the pads but the whole frame being raised, so that the datum line will be higher. Before supplying a narrower D.B.L., a frame of the required fitting must be tried to see if it is satisfactory. If it is found that the frame is raised sufficiently, then the narrower D.B.L. may be provided. If the frame is raised too much so that the datum line is too high with respect to the eyes, then this type of frame with its broad frontal angle is not suitable, and the client must be advised accordingly.

On the other hand, the situation may arise where the frame rests on the lower portion or even lower edge of the pads. It may not touch the nose on datum or at the top of the pads, as in Fig. 5.2.b. To provide a wider D.B.L. is seldom the answer in such a case. The difficulty is due to the frontal angle being too steep. A frame must be supplied with a greater frontal angle, and the D.B.L. checked again with the different type of frame.

Sometimes a different spread measurement may be possible, with the same eyesize and D.B.L., by using a keyhole instead of an arch pad fitting. The keyhole fitting provides a greater frontal angle and a greater control of spread measurements than the arch pad fitting.

Allowance must be made, however, for the fact that the person concerned may insist upon a frame of the style and appearance of Figs. 5.2a or 5.2b being supplied. In such cases, although the fittings shown may not be ideal, they do at least have the merit of positioning the frame correctly with respect to the eyes and as such may be the lesser of two evils. The optical effect of the lenses to be supplied will be correct, even if the frame is not perhaps as satisfactory or as comfortable as could be wished.

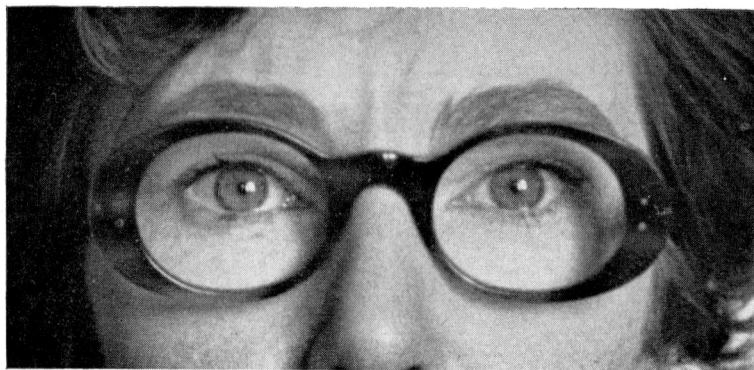
Fig. 5.3a. Frame too low on face. Regular bridge too high.

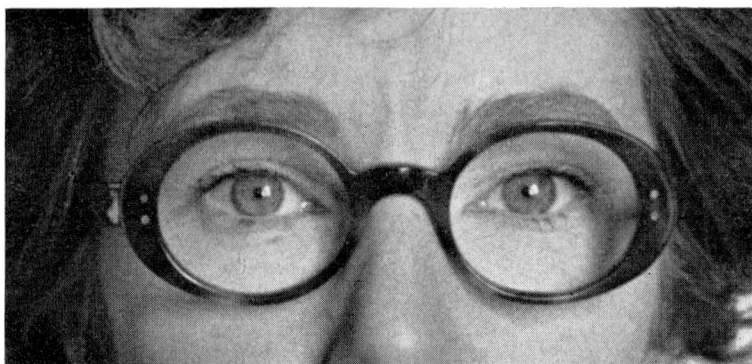
Fig. 5.3b. Bridge higher but frame still too low on face.

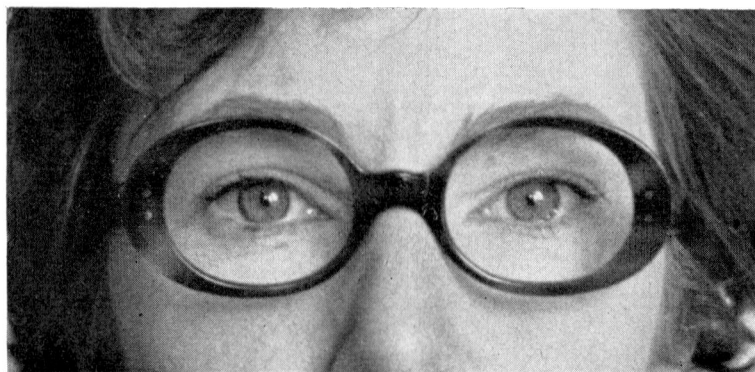
Fig. 5.3c. Frame correct on face.

76

(b) Regular bridge. Somewhat similar remarks apply to regular bridge fittings as to the above, except for observations about spread measurements.

Fig. 5.3a, b and c illustrate a series of frames which are respectively much too low, too low, and correct on the face.

The height of the bridge in Fig. 5.3a is 6 up, 5.3b is 3 up, and 5.3c is 0 up (i.e. on datum).

The spread of Fig. 5.3a is 14 @ 6 below crest, 5.3b is 13 @ 6, and 5.3c is 12 @ 6.

It will be seen that the frame in Fig. 5.3a is much too low on the face and requires to be raised, so the bridge height needs to be less. In Fig. 5.3b, the frame is still too low on the face and requires to be higher, so the bridge height must be less.

It should be noted that in each case, the spread measurement at a fixed position below crest remains almost the same, due allowance being made for the fact that the frame is fitted lower down in Fig. 5.3a than in 5.3b or 5.3c. The bridge of the frame rests on and around the bridge of the nose—this is what a regular bridge is intended for—so the spread measurement required will depend on the shape of the person's nose. In this respect it would be considered a facial rather than a frame measurement. This point is dealt with again in ¶6.8.

Having determined the spread measurement at 6 below crest, either by measurement from a frame which is nearly or exactly correct, or from a ruler with a set of spread measurements on it, the bridge height will then be determined by judgement from the nearest available fitting pattern. If the frame has to be raised relative to the pattern, than a lower bridge height will be required with a narrower dat. C.D. to give a slightly decreased spread at 6 below crest. If the frame has to be lowered relative to the pattern, then a higher bridge height will be required and a wider dat. C.D. to increase the spread slightly at 6 below crest. Greater judgement and experience are necessary with a regular bridge fitting than with a pad fitting.

The projection of either a pad bridge or a regular bridge will be determined by either the length of the lashes or the prominence of the cheeks or lids. Although the projection of the pad bridge is usually standard, some measure of control is often available by decreasing the D.B.L. This will lift the frame on the nose, so making it stand out from the face. The bridge fitting will then not fit the nose so comfortably, but will adapt the frame from an otherwise unsuitable or intolerable position.

For half-eye frames with regular bridge, much the same sort of considerations apply as to the above. However, there is one important difference. A half-eye frame is intended to fit lower down, so a fitting similar to that of Fig. 5.3a would enable the person to see over the top of the frame.

5.5. Supra Fitting

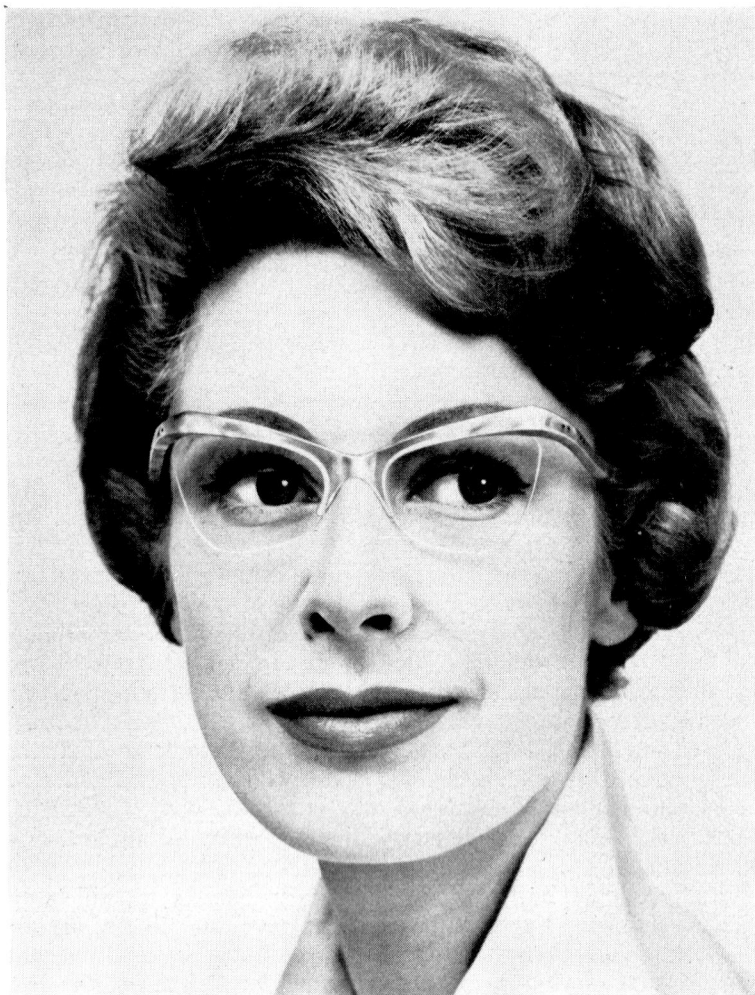

Fig. 5.4. Supra plastics frame, regular bridge.

The frame illustrated in Fig. 5.4 is a regular bridge supra style. The measurements are 44 × 34, 18 D.B.L., 5 up bridge, 12 @ 6.

If a deeper eyeshape is required, say 38, and glazed to this same frame, then the datum line will drop by 2 mm. (half the vertical difference). Consequently although the same frame is used, the bridge height will now be 7 up. This is an important point to keep in mind when fitting

78

supra frames. It also means that **all** measurements relative to the datum line, e.g. the "cut" of bifocal lenses, will be 2 mm. lower also.

If the datum line is to be brought back to its original position, the bridge height now required will be 5 up, relative to the new eyesize. However, a lower bridge with the same D.B.L. will result in a wider spread than the required 12 @ 6, probably 13 @ 6 or 14 @ 6. This, however, as previously explained, is a measurement that must be maintained to fit around the person's nose. So in addition to the bridge height being reduced, the D.B.L. will have to be reduced to bring the spread back to the required measurement.

All this sounds somewhat complicated, but with a little practice the dispenser will find himself able to deal with these situations, which become part of his normal work. The precise amount of allowance to make to the various measurements depend upon the circumstances pertaining to the case in hand.

5.6. Joint Position, Joint Angle, Temple Width and Length of Side

These various measurements have been included under one heading, as they are to some extent interdependent on one another. For example a centre joint position will need a shorter side than a high joint on an otherwise identical frame and on the same person, by some 5 – 7 mm.

The frame is fitted on the person, and the angle of joint observed.

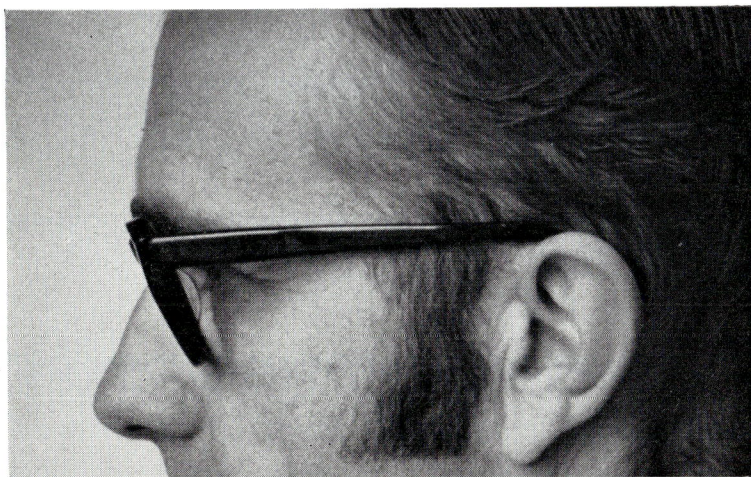

Fig. 5.5. Frame showing too great a joint angle.

In Fig. 5.5, a frame is illustrated which shows too great a joint angle. The angle is now $17\frac{1}{2}°$ and needs to be less by about 5°.

79

Whenever less angle is supplied, the joint will be moved nearer the ear, and a shorter side will be required. Conversely a greater joint angle will need a longer side.

The length of side is that length from the dowel pin (or joint screw) along the bottom of the side to the beginning of the bend, which should coincide with the top of the ear.

The angle of drop and splay of drop can be measured and specified, but are very easy to adjust in the finished spectacles. Length of drop is usually only necessary if something different (usually longer) is required. Otherwise a standard drop of about 30 mm. would be usual on a hockey end frame.

There are a number of frames which have a curl portion which is shaped around the ear. In this type, an overall length to include the curl portion will be needed. Such sides are usually supplied for children or athletics, where greater ability to hang on to the ear than the hockey end or straight sides is advocated. This type of side ensures a much firmer fit of the frame.

5.7. Metal Frames

Metal pad frames present little difficulty in measurement. They are, however, in very wide use throughout the world, and their country of origin should be noted. If the manufacturer in the country concerned uses the box system of measurement, and the frame is listed and probably stamped to this effect, then frames should likewise be measured and ordered using this system. Errors can arise from this cause. Usually the box lens size is larger than the datum lens size. So with a given dat. C.D., the D.B.L. will work out wrongly, or conversely, with a given D.B.L., the dat. C.D. will work out wrongly.

Metal W bridges are seldom used now, so it is not considered justified to give explanations as to how and in what way these frames should be measured and fitted. Reference to the list of measurements given under the heading of metal frames should probably be sufficient.

5.8. Adjustment

An important part of the fitting of spectacles is the final adjustment before the wearer takes them away, and also their continued adjustment to maintain the optimum comfort and lens efficiency.

It is extremely difficult to lay down any sort of procedure which may be followed in frame adjustment. So much will depend upon whether frame measurements were correct in the first place, whether they were correctly supplied by the works or Prescription House, whether the frame has warped in use (if plastics) or bent in use (if metal). So much will depend upon the wearer, for one person will tolerate and indeed request a frame which experience might suggest to be too wide or too narrow, too tight or too loose, and so on.

It is suggested therefore that spectacle adjustment cannot be taught at all from a book, but that it is essentially a practical art that can only be acquired by continual practice.

This begs the question and obviously is not very helpful, particularly to the student. But it is felt that only repeated practice will enable the art of spectacle adjustment to be acquired.

CHAPTER VI

FRAME STYLES

6.1. Historical Review

The topic of spectacle frame style is one which it is impossible to categorize. It cannot be stated that one certain style suits one certain person to the exclusion of all else. Perhaps the best way to demonstrate this is to look at the question of fashion from a historical point of view.

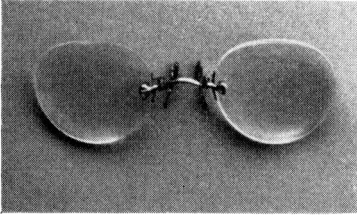

Fig. 6.1a. "F.P." mount.
1920

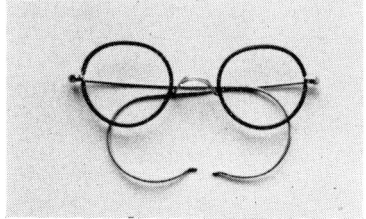

Fig. 6.1b. P.R.O. eye Windsor.
1930

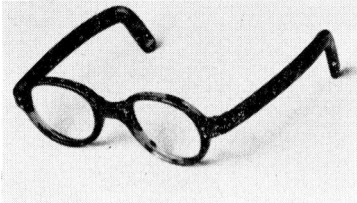

Fig. 6.1c. Heavy Library, regular bridge.
1940

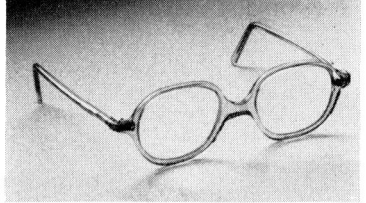

Fig. 6.1d. Light weight natural plastics.
1950

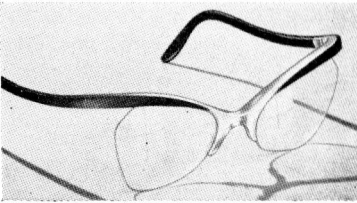

Fig. 6.1e. Acrylic supra.
1960

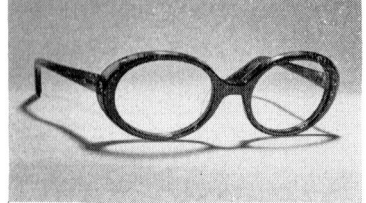

Fig. 6.1f. Large oval eye plastics.
1970

The above series of photographs is used to demonstrate the force of this argument. It would have been unthinkable in 1920 to supply anything except a Boston mount, an F.P. mount, or an oval eye metal frame. In fact the plastics materials that were to revolutionize the optical world in later decades had not been developed and produced.

Now in the latter half of the 20th century, it is unthinkable that such frames as were popular in 1920 could ever again acquire world-wide acceptance. What the future has to hold we cannot tell, but there is a definite trend in popularity for metal frames of the type shown below.

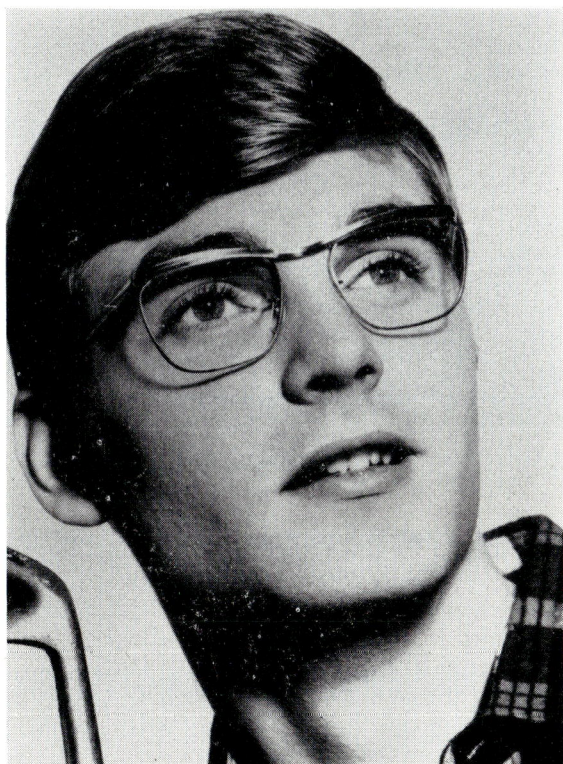

Fig. 6.2a. Metal pad frame.

Fig. 6.2a illustrates a metal pad bridge frame, and overleaf in fig. 6.2b is a metal combination frame. Both types of frame are popular in various forms.

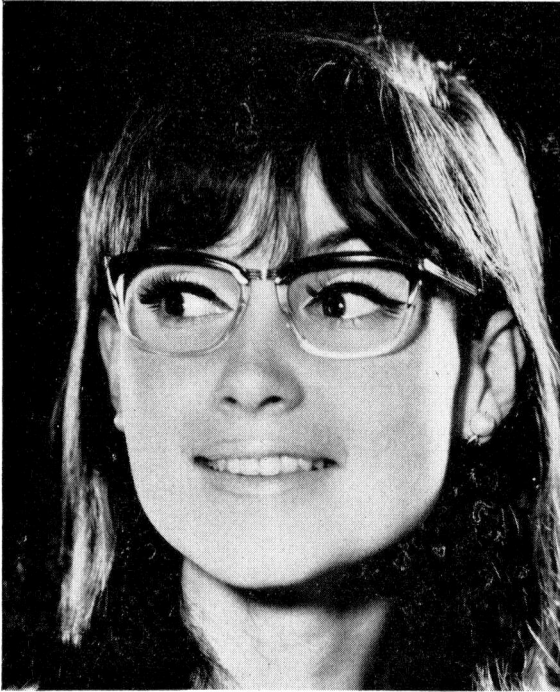

Fig. 6.2b. Metal combination frame.

It is therefore true to say that fashion is the dominating factor in frame styling. However, it will be found that as people grow older and one generation succeeds another, that the members of the preceding generation get set in their ideas, and tend with spectacle styles as with dress, to acquire a certain amount of rigidity in their outlook. They become less prepared to accept innovations, which tend to be the preserve of the young. So the older people are, the more "old-fashioned" their ideas and ideals in frame styles become.

The younger the optician and the younger the patient, the more "advanced" styling can be expected. The older the optician, the older the patient, the more "conservative" will be the style provided. However, all opticians should endeavour to keep up to date with the latest developments in frames and lenses. The patient comes to him for professional advice. It is the optician's responsibility to see that such advice is up to date.

6.2. Frame styling in Newspaper and Magazine Articles

Public figures in the world of entertainment, sport and politics, have a profound if not dominant influence upon the appearance of spectacles. Fashion designers and their models ensure that current ideas about frame styling are widely disseminated to the public. All these influences, much more than the advice which the optician offers, tend to make the choice of spectacle frames a matter of selection on the part of the patient.

The daily newspapers occasionally carry articles devoted to spectacles or spectacle frames. However, although infrequent, they do appear from time to time and with their immense readership of millions of people every day they obviously wield considerable influence.

The ladies' fashion magazines and the weekly periodicals also contain similar articles and these are much more frequent. In these cases, the articles on spectacle frames are often associated with advice on eye make-up, so it might perhaps be argued that opticians should become experts upon this also!

It is quite obvious from comments in practice that these articles reach a large number of people who ask for frames by the name of the person wearing a certain type of frame, or more usually describe in considerable detail the style of frame they have seen depicted. Unless the optician is aware of these styles, or of the immense influence wielded by the world of fashion particularly among ladies, he will not be able to meet the demands made upon him.

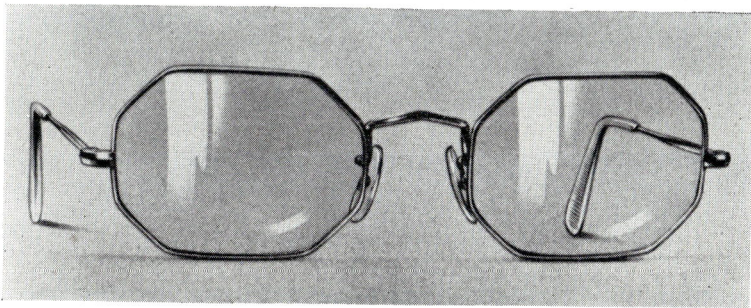

Fig. 6.3. "John Lennon" type spectacles.

The other main group of people who to a large extent come within the same category are the teenagers who are so largely influenced by their idols in the pop world. "John Lennon" spectacles are legendary, and Fig. 6.3. illustrates the type of frame which he first made famous. It should be noted however that the styles of frame that he has worn have varied somewhat over the years.

6.3. Frames for Ladies

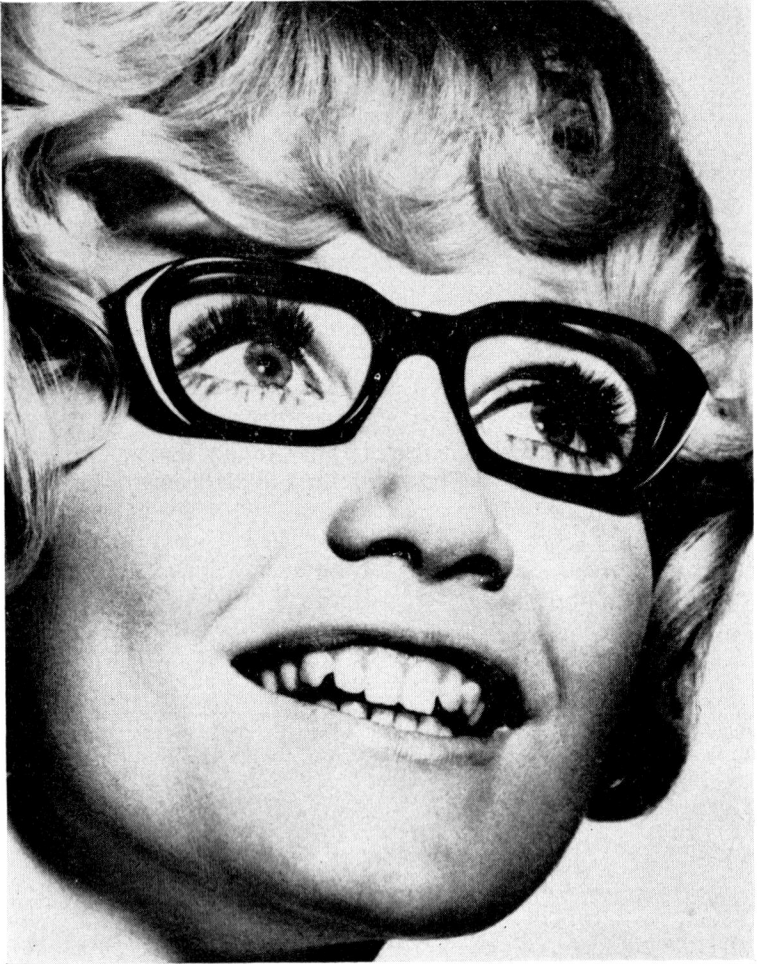

Fig. 6.4a. Round face, shallow eyeshape.

(a) Shape of face. How often one hears the plea "I want a pair of spectacle frames to suit me". And how difficult it is to advise the lady client just how this objective should best be achieved. Countless articles have been written primarily on the shape of the face, for this is the factor which appears most to influence the choice.

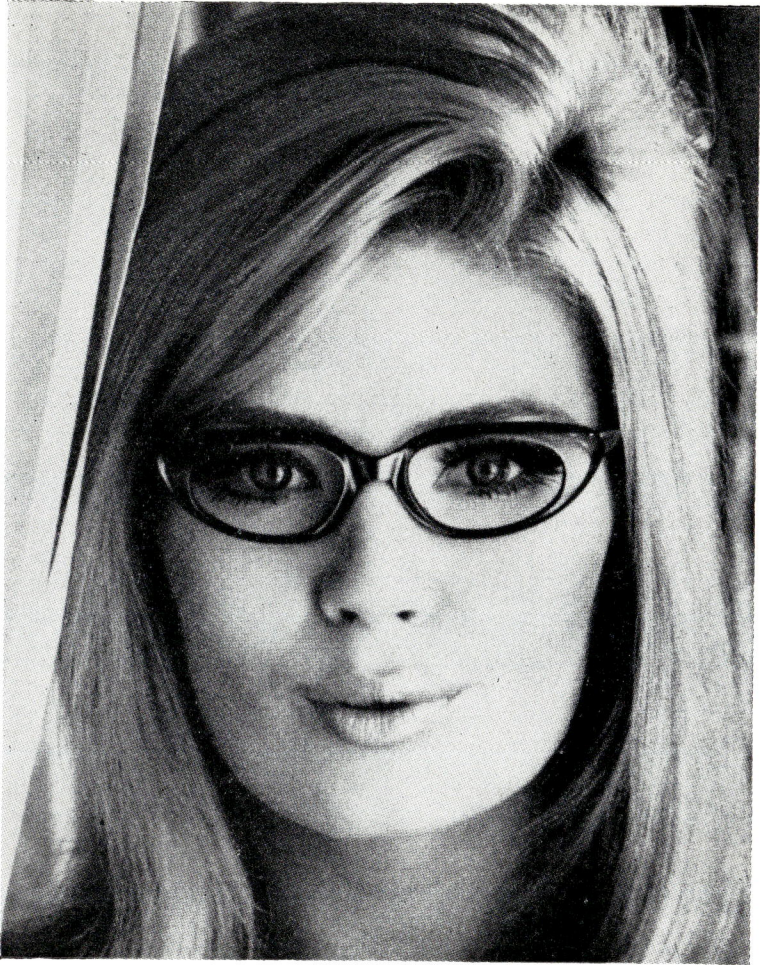

Fig. 6.4b. "Square" face, shallow eyeshape although a little more upswept

It is generally accepted that in the absence of any other complicating circumstances, that a round face, Fig 6 4a, or a "square" face, Fig. 6.4b, should have a shallow lens shape; the lack of depth of the lens and the elongating effect (especially of somewat pointed frame-temples), helping to detract attention from and to offset the roundness of the face or fullness of the jaw. Furthermore, the shallow shape avoids the frame sitting on the cheeks.

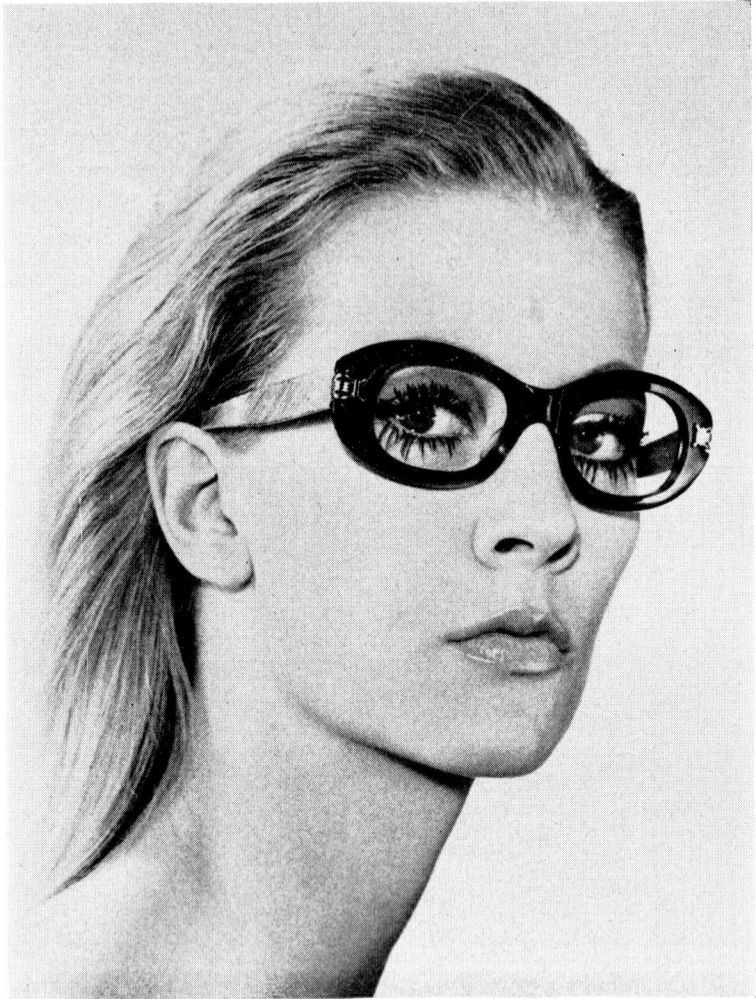

Fig. 6.4c. Oval face, more rounded and somewhat deeper eyeshape.

In Fig. 6.4c, the oval face, exactly the opposite effect needs to be achieved. The face needs to be "filled out" by making the lenses a little deeper or rounder than in Figs. 6.4a or 6.4b, and with the frame-temples less pronounced or pointed, possibly by having the joints more nearly central. This shape has often been described as the "perfect" face, and its possessor is fortunate in being able to wear almost any style and still look nice.

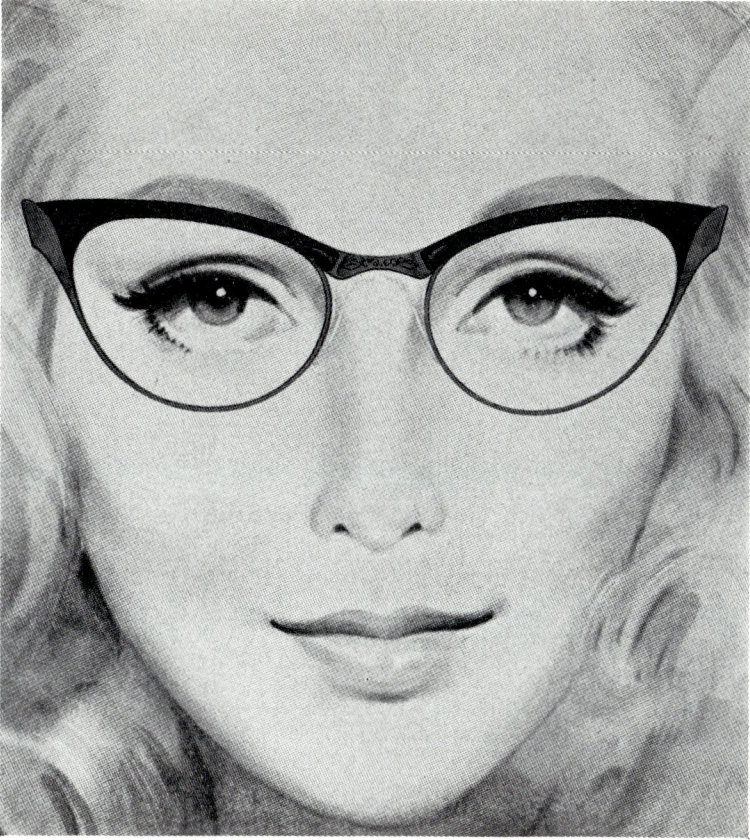

Fig. 6.4d. Pointed or longer face, upswept lens shape.

In the pointed (or longer) face, Fig. 6.4d, it is probable that a frame which is of the "upswept" shape is best, as this appears to conform to the facial contours, and takes attention away from the temples and forehead which are disproportionately wide as compared with the balance of the face.

This approach, based on the shape of the person's face, is a rewarding one, for it offers something tangible about which the optician is able to advise his client.

It is, however, only a small part of a very big whole and must be limited primarily to ladies who are fashion conscious.

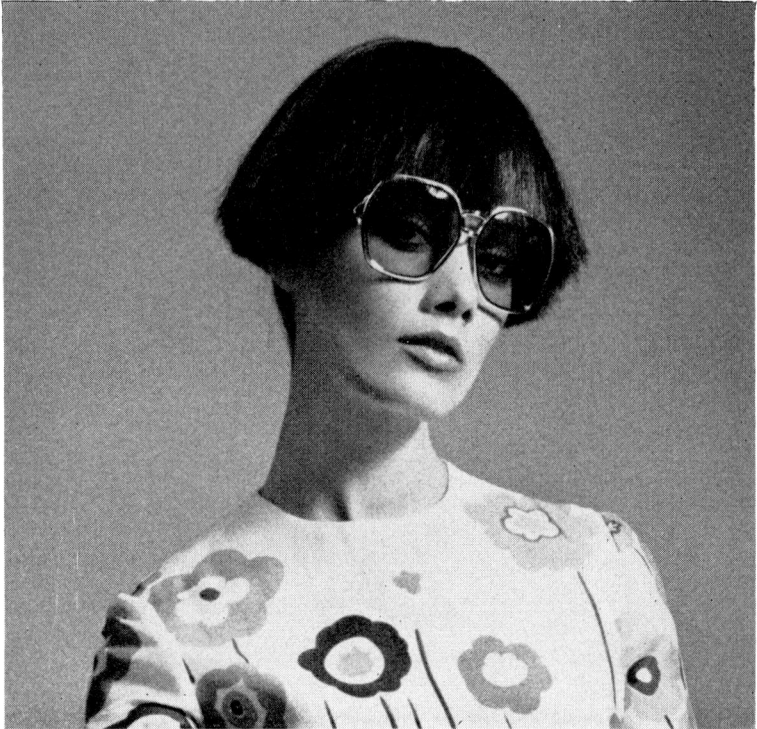

Fig. 6.5a. Large almost round eyeshape.

(b) Age of person. Adult spectacle wearers may be split up into the following age groups:-

    (i)   teenagers, say 15 – 20.
    (ii)   age 20 – 45.
    (iii) age 45 – 65.
    (iv) age over 65.

It must be realized that the following remarks are only generalisations, and do not apply to every case.

(i) Teenagers usually require the most "with-it" style, which may vary from year to year quite sharply. The very large lenses are the fashion of the early 1970s. These may be round or roundish, Fig. 6.5a, or angular, Fig. 6.5b. Eventually as the teenagers grow up and grow older, they will either bring their own styles into the later age group, or adopt the styles of the somewhat older person.

90

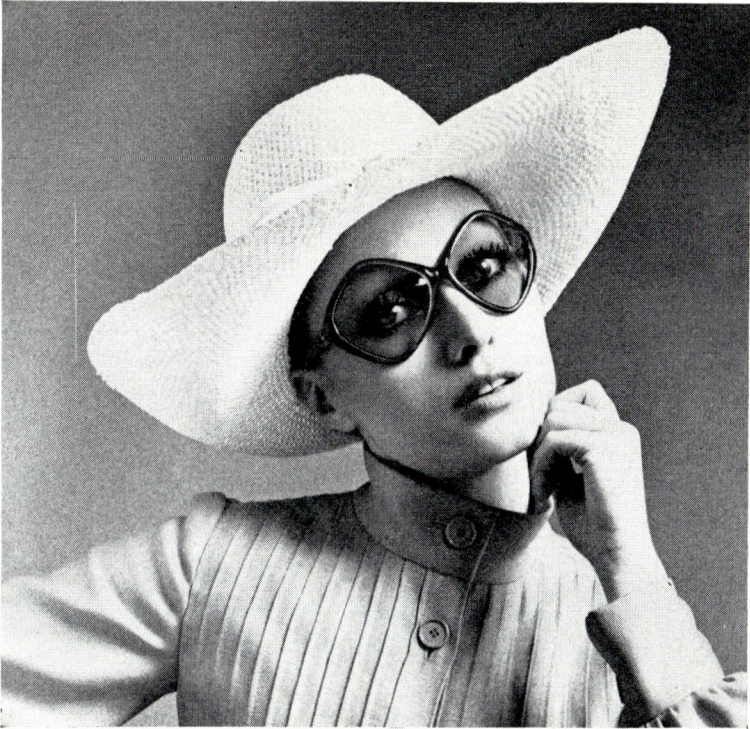

Fig. 6.5b. large angular eyeshape.

Observation of the current sunglass styles will usually provide a very fair indication of what next year's fashions are likely to be for this younger age group.

There will of course always be a certain element of older people who like the younger styles also, and will at least ask to see them and to try them.

(ii) Age group 20 – 45. These persons are the ones most likely to be influenced by fashion considerations such as those described and illustrated in Figs. 6.4a to Fig. 6.4d.

(iii) Age group 45 – 65. We now have the more conservative age group, still conscious of their appearance and wishing to look their best in glasses, but who will not accept very readily the advent of the more recent styles. Advice to these people must revolve around styles which have been popular for some little time.

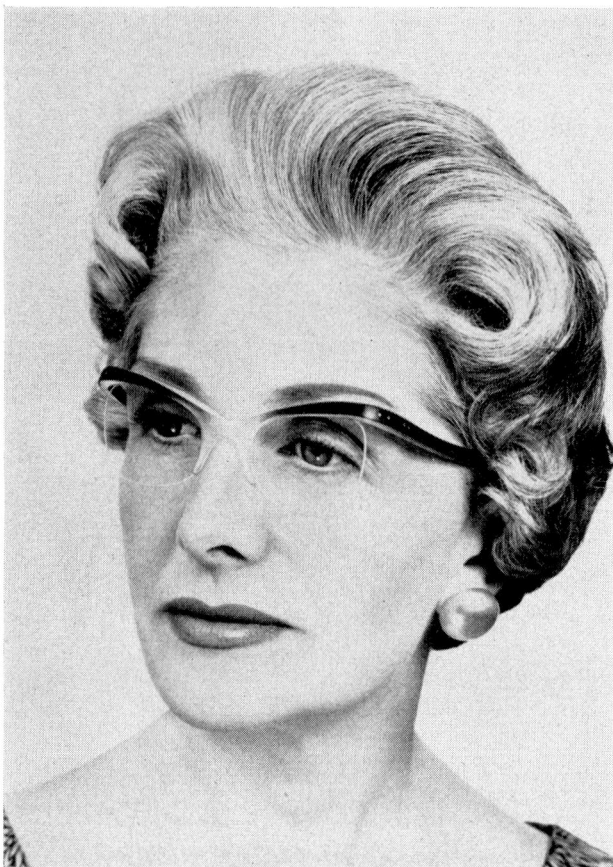

Fig. 6.6a. Supra style on older face.

It must be remembered that older people have faces which tend to be rounder and fuller than younger people, and deeper lens shapes are more acceptable on this account. Also we are now dealing with presbyopes needing either reading glasses only, or bifocals or multifocals. In either event, as the eyes will have to be directed downwards to look at reading matter in the lower field of vision, the deeper shape is an optical necessity.

The supra style, Fig. 6.6a, in particular has much to recommend it for this age group. It is usually more youthful looking as it softens the line of the older face with its heavier cheeks and jowls.

92

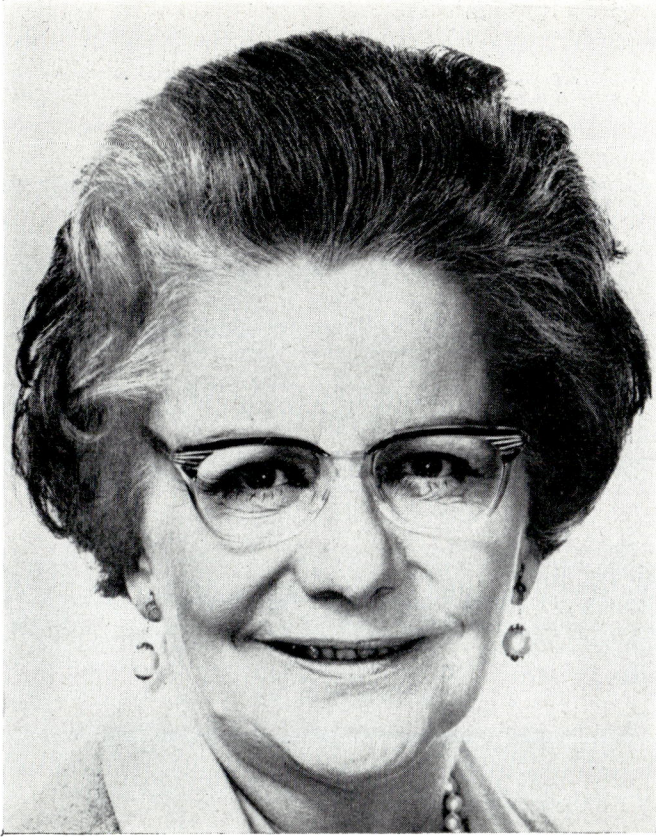
Fig. 6.6b. Two-tone frame on older face.

Attention in Fig. 6.6a is obviously directed upwards to the frame at the expense of the rimless lower portion, and this gives an upswept effect. This may be further enhanced by making the frame or lens slightly upswept also.

However it should not be assumed that supra styles are only suitable for older people, as this is by no means the case. Supras are very suitable indeed in many cases for younger people. They are lighter in weight, and much lighter in appearance.

A similar effect could have been achieved by a two-tone frame, Fig. 6.6b, with a dark or coloured top and a transparent lower portion.

(iv) Age over 65. Generally speaking ladies in this age group are not so conscious of their appearance, and as long as the styling is not too functional they are fairly easy to please.

(c) Smartness of person. In all age groups, the styling of the hair, the shape of the eyebrows (which may in any case be altered as required with ladies), the shape and length of the nose, the shape of the mouth and chin, the fullness of the mouth and cheeks, and all the other factors which go to make up the appearance of a person's face must obviously be taken into consideration.

In this respect, an important factor is the smartness or elegance of the lady. This is an imponderable quality which defies description, but to supply a dowdy person with a smart frame, or a smart person with a dowdy frame, is a faux-pas to be avoided at all costs. There might perhaps be some justification in trying to make a person who is drab and dreary look more attractive, but to make an attractive person look less so by unbecoming spectacles is a disaster. To advise the person solely on the shape of the face, or age, and irrespective of any other factor, is not therefore to be advocated.

(d) Evening wear. Slowly and gradually, the concept of glasses for special occasions is gradually being accepted. This is a different matter from the question of a "spare" pair as a hedge against breakage or emergency. See ¶1.2 & ¶6.8.

In particular, the major occasions upon which ladies wear their jewellery and their most elegant dresses are for social events, usually in the evenings. A decorated or more fancy pair of frames is a great advantage.

6.4. Frames for Men

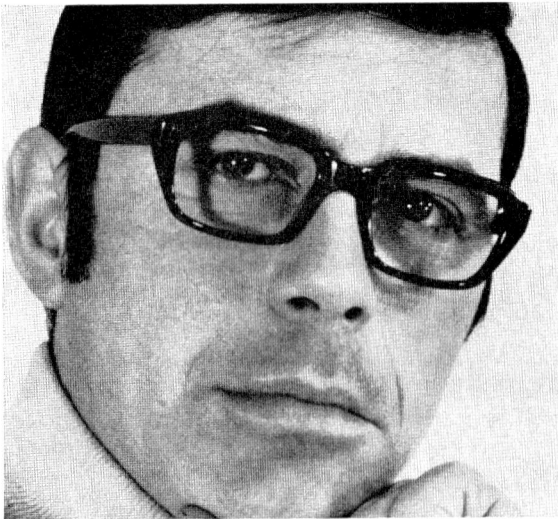

Fig. 6.7a. Heavy weight frame, robust features.

94

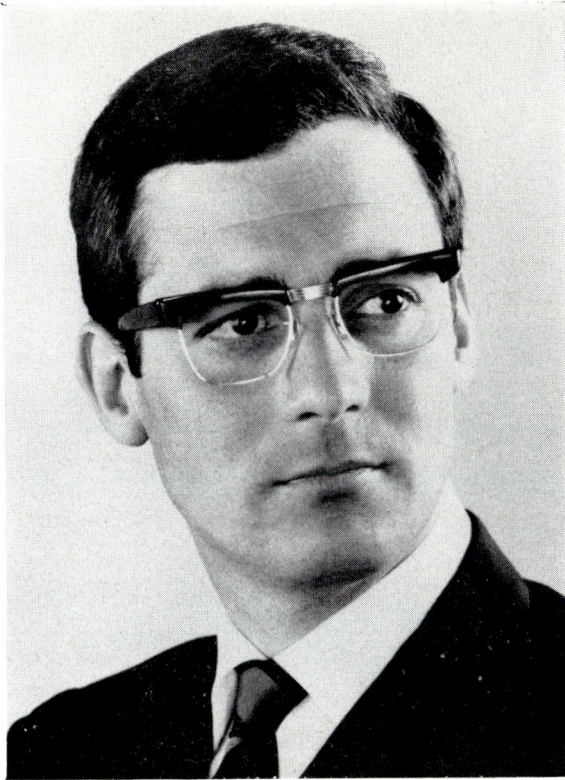

Fig. 6.7b. Lighter weight frame, more slender build.

It seems by tacit consent in the case of men, not to be so much a matter of the shape of the face, as the lightness or heaviness of the build of the face. A heavy face, Fig. 6.7a, requires a full frame, substantial and solid. A more slender face, Fig. 6.7b, requires a lighter weight frame.

The average human male is bigger and heavier in build than the average human female. He undertakes heavier work. He is more liable to damage his spectacles through accident or wear and tear. To this extent, therefore, it is usual for most men to have spectacle frames which are rather more robust or physically stronger than those in use for ladies.

The optician must beware if there is a history of migraine, sinus trouble, or some other factor which militates against the use of anything which will cause pressure upon the nerves of the region of the upper face. Inevitably spectacles must rest on the skin of the nose, so if it is suspected or implied that there are difficulties of this nature, then the major consideration above all must be the lightness of weight of spectacles (both frame and lenses) which are supplied.

95

6.5. Frames for Children

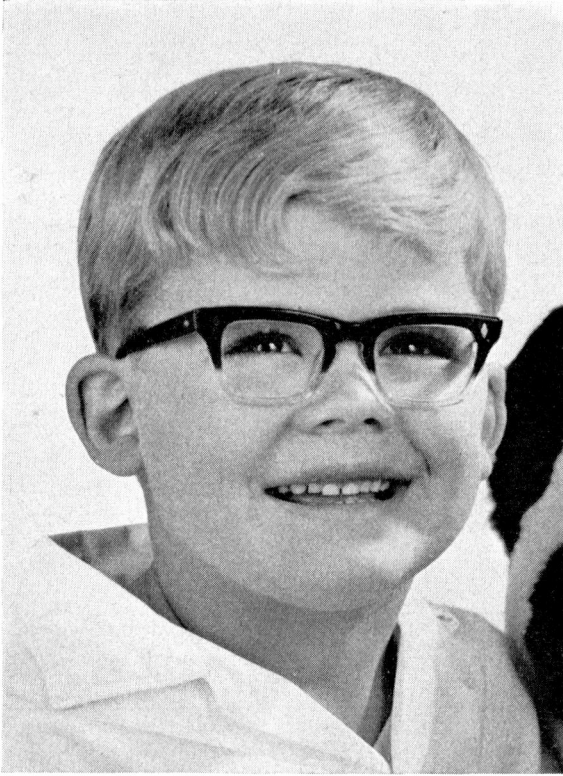

Fig. 6.8a. Children's combination frame.

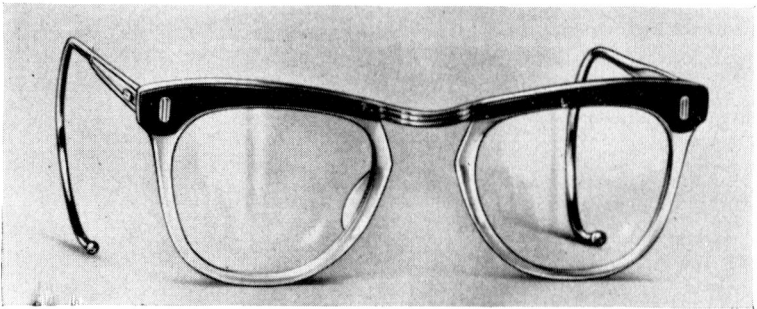

Fig. 6.8b. Childrens' plastics frame.

It is invariably found that children have much less pronounced bridges to their noses than adults, so regular bridges are never used for this purpose. The practice is to supply either metal or metal combination pad frames Fig. 6.8a, or plastics pad frames Fig. 6.8b. Different manufacturers with different frames will attempt to shape the pad or the spread or the frontal angle of the frame to adapt it to the different shaped nose from that found in adults, and the frame illustrated in Fig. 6.8b above has a slightly different curved and shaped pad from that usually fitted to adults' frames.

6.6. Frame Styles in Foreign Countries

The foregoing remarks applying to frame styles for men, women and children are not universal in application. Patterns, styles and even materials vary widely from country to country in different parts of the world.

Other countries of the world where social benefit schemes are in existence which are similar to those found in Gt. Britain, may or may not have regulations which are as restrictive as those found here, The strictures which apply to lens shapes, methods of mounting, etc., obviously have an adverse effect upon free choice of what might otherwise be considered to be the most suitable style for a particular person.

The material of which the frame is made has an important bearing, for undoubtedly the most popular man's frame on the Continent of Europe is the metal or metal combination pad frame. This is not so widely used in Britain. A heavier pattern plastics frame, monotone or two-tone, is much more customary. It is impossible to determine any reason for this.

In the United States of America, the most popular ladies' frame is the metal combination, usually with pads, and the metal very often is aluminium alloy. Such frame styles are little worn in Europe.

The variation of frame styles and even of frame materials, from country to country, is a fascinating reflection of national characteristics and likes and dislikes.

6.7. Colour of Frames

During the period 1955 – 1965, chiefly due to the introduction of acrylic materials which could take brilliant colours in a vast array and which were reasonably "fast", i.e. would not fade, coloured frames became very popular with ladies. However, the last five years of the 1960s saw the introduction of heavier black or dark coloured frames, which became all the rage. Then in the early 1970s black became much less popular and various shades of brown, mottled, and light mottled plastics very largely took the place of the black. Much more could be written about this topic, but it is felt that a text-book intended to last for a number of years is not the appropriate place. This book is designed for students and trainees as well as established opticians, and the object is to attempt to lay down general principles. With fashions changing as fast as they do in modern times, what is current fashion in one period of time will most certainly not be so in 10 or even 5 years, as has been demonstrated when discussing colours.

Discussion about the individual merits of particular features such as colour and shape is best left to the optical press, to fashion houses, to designers, to frame manufacturers, and all the various other interested parties who may be concerned in any way with the changing optical scene.

6.8. Frame Size

There is one aspect of frame fashion, however, which most definitely influences the measurements necessary for frames and this is the size of the lenses. Mention has already been made of the size of supra lenses and the bridge heights that must be noted in this context (see ¶5.5 and see also Ch. 7).

In particular, the bridge fittings supplied to the normal range of frames are based upon an **average** of face and nose shapes. If a style or size is required which is very different from the norm, it will be found very often that an average size of fitting will no longer be possible.

The problem is illustrated by the two photographs in Fig. 6.9.a and b.

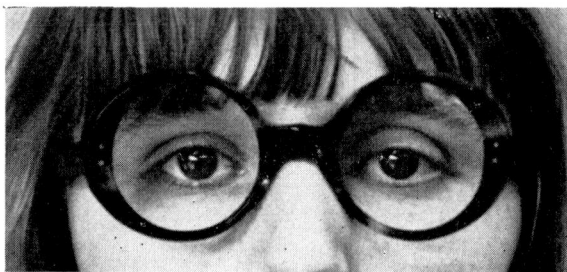

Fig. 6.9a. Regular bridge, reasonable fitting.

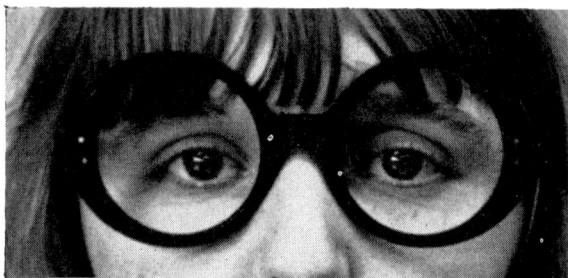

Fig. 6.9b. Regular bridge, same measurements as Fig. 6.9a, poor fitting.

98

Fig. 6.9a shows a nicely fitted frame, regular bridge plastics, 44 × 66, 22 D.B.L., 2 × 2, 14 @ 6 below crest (front measurement only). It fits nicely around the contours of the nose, positions the lenses well with regard to the pupils of the eyes, and should be satisfactory in use.

Fig. 6.9b shows a 50 × 72 frame, and the bridge measurements are exactly the same as in Fig. 6.9a, being 22 D.B.L., 2 × 2, 14 @ 6. However it will be noticed that the bearing surface of the frame is now on the side of the nose and the cheeks. The datum line has been thrown much too high, the eyebrows are too visible within the lenses. Generally the frame is unsatisfactory and will be uncomfortable in use.

The point to be emphasized is that **the bridge fitting is the same** in the two frames. In order to provide a large lens size frame as in Fig. 6.9b, the bridge needs to be lower, and the D.B.L. wider.

It is wrong therefore to assume that having measured a person for a certain frame that this measurement is correct for all other sizes and styles. This is the main criticism levelled at attempting to measure a subject from a set of rulers. The fit of the individual frame is all-important, and what is correct for one case is not necessarily correct for another. Fig 6.9b is an exaggerated case, but the principle is sound. It applies equally to pad bridge frames and regular bridge frames.

Having posed the question its solution is not so simple, for it will depend on the style required. Few frames are of the large size illustrated by Fig. 6.9b, so the difference between the frames is not likely to be so great as that shown here.

In general, however, the example merely serves to emphasize the principle that it is essential to have a sample frame which is as nearly like the finished article required as possible, so that a reasonable estimate may be made by the optician of any slight amendments to the measurements that may be required.

It might be observed once again that the importance of the frontal angle of the frame is important in this context. Reference to this has already been made in ¶4.4 when discussing measurement (xiii) of a pad frame. It has also been discussed in ¶5.4.

6.9. Functional Dispensing

Here the optician comes more fully into his own. When required for a specific purpose, the selection of frame style or lens shape or position on the face, etc., is not so much a matter of individual choice or so much at the whim of fashion or fancy.

Spectacles are worn for the following purposes:-
- (a) general use.
- (b) distance use only.
- (c) reading use only (or for other close wear purposes, and invariably associated with presbyopia).
- (d) bifocal or multifocal use.

Spectacles which are intended to be used for purpose (a) are the usually accepted standard by which the frames are fitted on the face, and for which they are measured. The measurements listed in Chapter 4 are based on this fact. This position of the frames constitutes a compromise between the position necessary for (b) and (c).

If spectacles are to be used for purpose (b), they should in general be fitted a little higher on the face, and with a little less joint angle, so that the wearer looks more normally through the lenses when his gaze is directed straight ahead.

If spectacles are to be fitted for purpose (c), they should be fitted a little lower on the face, with a little more joint angle. Again the object is to enable the wearer to look more normally through the lenses when the line of fixation passes through a point further down the lens surface. This is so that the prismatic effect due to the effective decentration is as little as possible (it should be apparent that since the eye looks through the lens at a point below the optical centre, this constitutes an effective decentration).

Spectacles worn for purpose (d) represent the most difficult aspect of the technique of frame fitting. One important matter must be borne in mind throughout. It is easier to change the **frame** than it is to change the **lenses,** if there is any query or complaint about the positioning of them. For example, if the patient complains that he can see the dividing line of the bifocal when looking straight ahead or when walking about, it is easier to supply a new frame which will drop the datum line relative to the person's eyes, rather than to supply a new pair of lenses in which the bifocal segment is cut lower (the "cut" being the depth below datum of the segment top).

Experience teaches that bifocals (or multifocals) need a deeper lens shape than single sight lenses. Also they need to be fitted a little lower on the face than constant wear spectacles—assuming that the bifocals (or multifocals) are of such a correction that the distance portion is for constant use. Some bifocals, however, are worn for convenience where the top portion is plano or with a minor correction, and the segment portion is by far the more important. This is the sort of bifocal (or multi-focal) where the person does not want to have to keep putting on and taking off a presbyopic reading correction. In such cases, the spectacles should be fitted fairly high on the face, and the cut positioned high in the frame also, so the maximum use may be made of the bifocal segment area.

It would appear that there is a vastly greater potential for half-eye spectacles than is currently in vogue for purpose (c). Certainly they have been popularized by certain public figures, chiefly in the political field.

6.10. Alternative pairs of spectacles for various purposes

Mention has been made of the purposes for which spectacles are required under the headings (a), (b), (c) and (d). However, this is the most obvious of the categories into which spectacles for different purposes could be grouped, and makes no provision whatever for the fact that each individual differs from his neighbour in his optical requirements. Our previous sub-divisions are dependent upon the onset and degree of presbyopia, but social behaviour, type of work, working fixation distance, sport, possibility of damage, age of subject etc., all receive some acknowledgement at times, but not as much as they should.

Functional dispensing is still regarded by some as unprofessional. This attitude of mind regards an optician's responsibilities as limited to supplying such spectacles or optical appliances as he is specifically requested to do by his patient. However the patient usually knows little or nothing about specialist ophthalmic services, and frames and particularly lenses are a mystery about which he seeks advice and information. Most opticians would carry out their function more adequately if they were to explain in greater detail the alternatives available. In this sense, "spare" pairs become "alternative" pairs and the patient is better served optically.

6.11. Attempts to Introduce Rationalisation into Frame Fitting

Many attempts have been made from time to time to try and formulate principles whereby a system or systems of frame measurements and styling may be determined. Mr. L. S. Sasieni's two books have already been referred to in the preface.

Mention should be made of the various articles on cosmetic dispensing from the pen of Mr. W. S. Topliss, B.O.A. (Disp.), S.M.C. (Disp.), which have appeared in *The Optician* on various occasions; vide November 25, 1966 and March 22/29, 1968, in particular.

These are only two authors amongst many who have tried to insert some sort of system into a rather chaotic situation. It is perhaps unfair to mention these to the exclusion of all others, but they have each tried a different approach, and under certain circumstances each system will have its advantages and adherents.

It is hoped that more direction will be applied towards investigation into these topics and related matters. This could well form the basis of research projects in Universities and Colleges which have optics departments.

CHAPTER VII

INFLUENCE OF LENSES UPON FRAME STYLES

7.1. Size of Lens

Most of the remarks made during the preceding chapters apply with equal validity to this chapter also, with one very important reservation. Most lenses which differ from what might be termed the "ordinary" or usual range of single-sight lenses, say up to ± 3.00D sphere with cylindrical powers of up to ± 2.00D, are available in stock blanks up to 50 – 55 mm. in diameter. This does not apply to all lens manufacturers, or to all powers, and for precise details of sizes the reader is referred to the catalogues of the manufacturer concerned or to a Prescription House from whom enquiries may be made.

Further complications arise from the fact that lens blank sizes are often not circular, even stock blanks being "square", i.e. rectangular with rounded corners. Where cylinders are worked on them, they are normally made with the axis parallel to a flat edge. If the finished Rx calls for an oblique axis and an asymmetrical shape is required (particularly if it is an upswept shape), then the final edging from the lens blank is quite a complicated matter.

7.2. Decentration

The question of decentration also enters materially into these considerations. When calculating the maximum size of centred lens blank from which a certain lens may be cut or edged, the rule is:- centred lens blank size = finished lens size + 2 (decentration) + edging allowance.

O is the optical and geometrical centre of the round lens blank shown in Fig. 7.1. A shallow PRO (panto round-oval) lens shape is shown superimposed on it, such that the datum line of the lens passes through O. d is the amount of decentration available on each side of the lens shape. If for instance the lens blank size is 54 mm., and the lens shape is 46 mm. horizontally, then the maximum available amount of decentration will be 4 mm. each side, less the edging allowance. $1 - 1\frac{1}{2}$ mm. is usually allowed each side for glazing, so the maximum amount of decentration is therefore finally $2\frac{1}{2} - 3$ mm.

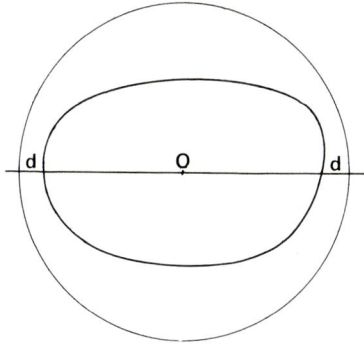

Fig. 7.1. Shallow P.R.O. lens shape superimposed on round lens blank.

7.3. Shape Wastage Factor

An attempt to overcome the difficulties dealt with above by establishing a rule which will enable minimum lens blank sizes to be determined for different asymmetrical shapes, involves the concept of the **Shape Wastage Factor.**

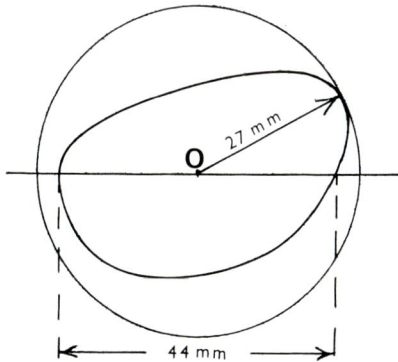

Fig. 7.2a. Upswept lens shape superimposed on round lens blank. O is the optical centre of the blank, and coincides with the datum centre of the lens shape.

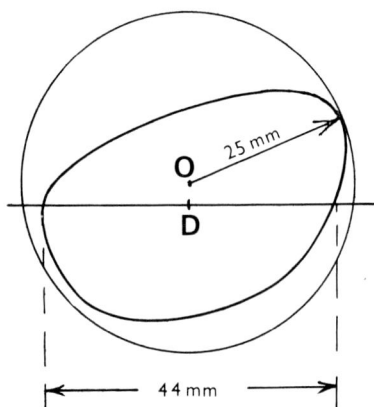

Fig. 7.2b. Upswept lens shape superimposed on round lens blank. O is the optical centre of the blank, and D is the datum centre of the lens shape.

Fig. 7.2a shows an upswept shape which has a long diameter of 27 mm. from O, the optical and geometrical centre of the blank. O also coincides with the datum centre of the finished lens shape. It is obvious from the diagram that a 54 mm. blank (allowing nothing for edging) will be needed to permit this lens shape to be obtained. The datum length however is only 44 mm. The difference between the uncut lens size and the horizontal datum length is the S.W.F., being 54 – 44 = 10 mm. in this case. The smaller the S.W.F., the more symmetrical is the lens shape.

Another way of reducing the uncut lens size for any given shape is to position the optical centre a little above the datum centre (no decentration or prism being present), by positioning the finished lens size lower on the original blank. Fig. 7.2b shows this for the upswept shape previously considered. In this case, O is 3 mm. above D (datum centre of finished lens shape), needing only about 50 mm. lens blank. There is now therefore 4 mm. more material to work with, allowing greater decentration to be given for the same size lens and same size uncut. This is an obvious advantage, and is one of the reasons why most Prescription Houses position the O.C. above the datum centre as previously referred to.

In addition to this upward decentration, it should be clear from the diagram 7.2b that an even smaller uncut could be used if the lens is decentred outwards as well. This is of particular importance when heavy lenses (e.g. aphakic corrections) are needed and when it is necessary to keep uncut and lens sizes to a minimum. This outward decentration also permits the supply of a frame dat. C.D. less than the P.D. but with accurately centred lenses.

7.4. Difficulties in Dispensing Large Lenses

When a patient requests a large lens size, (a tendency noticable for many years), considerations such as the above that have been discussed in ¶7.1 to ¶7.3, immediately assume large proportions. The patient may for instance require the following Rx:-

R. +3.00 / +1.00 × 140 : L. +4.00 / +2.00 × 70

The finished datum lens size may be requested to be 50 mm., the frame dat. C.D. needs to be 72 mm., and the P.D. of the person is 62 mm. for distance. A quick mental calculation shows that the decentration required is 5 mm. in each eye, so that a lens blank size of 50 + 2(5) + 3 = 63 mm. would be necessary. This is greater than is available. In fact, it is doubtful if any manufacturer has a stock lens blank of greater than 50 mm. for the L.E. It is possible to obtain the decentration required by working a prism on the lens, but whilst optically satisfactory, it would be quite impractical as it would be so heavy, besides being cosmetically objectionable.

It is therefore necessary to advise such a person that the 50 mm. lens size which he requires cannot be obtained to his prescription and requirements. This is a matter which arises very often, and it needs considerable practice on the part of the optician to be able to advise his patient quickly as to what type, size, shape and style of frame he **cannot** have.

It is considered that this is one of the most important functions of the dispensing of spectacles by an optician. It is useless showing or discussing with patients large numbers of different frame styles, if many of them are not capable of being used anyway. There are technical barriers which automatically arise to prevent a completely free choice being exercised. The good dispenser will know what these barriers are, and from practice he will know to a large extent what frame sizes and styles to eliminate so as not to prolong the discussion or complicate it unnecessarily —or even to prevent future difficulty when patients return complaining of discomfort, or constant slipping, or one of the many other troubles that are experienced.

Broadly speaking, it is best technically to err on the side of smallness of size, lightness of weight and comfort in wear. Unfortunately this conflicts diametrically with the requirements of the patient who nearly always wants as large a lens size as possible. Alternatively, the frame style required may only be available in large eyesizes. The two objectives are often incompatible, and the optician must exercise his judgement as to where to effect the best compromise.

Many examples could be given of how difficulties of the general pattern discussed throughout ¶7.1 to ¶7.4 may be solved, but almost every case present its own peculiarities. Practice and experience is really the only means of enabling the optician to solve them.

7.5. Frames Necessary for High-Power Lenses

In particular this concerns spectacles to be supplied to (a) aphakic patients (i.e. the crystalline lens of the eye is missing usually as a result of a cataract operation), and (b) to patients who need a myopic correction in excess of say —12.00D sph.

(a) High-Power Positive Lenses. Many patients complain of the weight of lenses even when only +3.00D sph., particularly if a large size lens requiring decentration is used. How much more difficult this problem is therefore when the patient needs a +12.00D sph. lens (with usually a cyl. correction up to +3.00D axis approx. 180°). If dispensed as a full-aperture glass lens, the size **must** be kept to a minimum, exaggerated shapes avoided, and decentration allowed only to the extent that the uncut size is at a minimum, otherwise the weight will prove to be too heavy for both comfort and practicability. The spectacles will be uncomfortable in use and will in all probability slip down the nose, so preventing the correct optical effect being achieved.

The alternative is a full-aperture plastics lens (which seems by far the best alternative), or a plastics lenticular. In both these cases, the bulbous effect of the greater curvature on the front surface of the plastics lenses will cause more scratching than with glass. However, larger lens sizes may be supplied, up to the blank size available. Alternatively, glass lenticulars in one of several forms may be supplied also, with larger lens sizes if necessary.

Summing up, therefore, we have the following alternatives for lenses which may be supplied for a high-power positive correction.

    (i)   full aperture glass (flat or toric).

    (ii) full aperture plastics.

    (iii) glass lenticulars, in solid, uniseal or cement methods.

    (iv) plastics lenticulars.

(i) has much to recommend it. It is relatively cheap; it gives with (ii) the widest field of view possible with an aphakic correction (which is an enormous advantage to the wearer); it is fairly quick to obtain compared with (ii), (iii) or (iv); it is the least likely to suffer damage due to scratching. Its disadvantage is weight, so a smaller lens size is advisable than with the other types.

(ii) has the advantage of lighter weight than (i), so a larger lens size may be employed. However, it is more steeply curved on the front surface than even the toric form of (i) due to the less refractive index of the material. This factor together with the fact that the plastics substance is softer, means that the lens is more easily scratched.

(iii) both glass and plastics lenticulars have the disadvantage of making an already reduced field of view even smaller than full-aperture lenses. However, to compensate for this they have the enormous advantage of lightness of weight. Solid, uniseal or cement segments may be supplied.

The optical performance of these different types is much the same, but the methods of production vary. The segments may be on the inside or outside of the lens, If on the outside, it conforms more nearly to best-form theory, but is mechanically not so good.

(iv) lenticulars of plastics material are the lightest of all, but besides the reduction in the field of view already referred to, this lens is the most easily scratched of the four types.

In all these cases we are not discussing the technical performance of the lenses. The optics of the problem is not our concern at the moment. We are only interested in the dispensing and supply of the frames into which such lenses have to be fitted, and their subsequent behaviour. Two main matters which are interconnected are under consideration, therefore: these are the size and weight of the lenses.

(b) High-Power Negative Lenses. There are various ways of dealing with prescriptions which call for high-power negative lenses, and these may consist of special edging techniques, such as "mini-bevelling"; of having lenticular portions worked on the lenses; or having the surfaces and/or edges anti-reflection coated, etc. The variety of methods of dealing with such prescriptions is much greater than the alternatives available with high-power positive lenses, so it is not deemed advisable to go too deeply into these matters here. Suffice it to say that particularly when dealing with lenticulars, whether convex-flattened, myotor, profiled, or one of the several other types, the lens size **must** be kept fairly small. Most wearers are acutely conscious of the appearance of minus lenticular lenses and object strongly to the circular or shaped central portion showing too much (or having too small a lenticular portion), or showing too many internal reflections in the form of "power-rings". Certainly the best way of dealing with this is to keep to as small a lens size as practical, so using the frame as camouflage to hide the thickness of lens.

One important matter has been left until the end of this discussion of lens and frame sizes for high-power lenses. When referring to a large lens size or a small lens size, we invariably mean the horizontal diameter, not the vertical. It is sometimes thought that because a lens shape is shallow, i.e. 44 × 30 oval or shallow P.R.O., that such a lens size may be increased without giving rise to difficulties due to size. However, whilst it is true that such a lens looks small as compared with say a 44 × 40 quadra, this is an optical illusion and the horizontal diameter is the same. It has to be cut from the same size lens blank, and needs the same decentration horizontally when fitted to the same person in the same D.B.L. frame. In fact, shallow lens shapes when edged from toric blanks of high-power give rise to many other troubles due to the shape of the V-edging, and the distortion that has to be deliberately effected (in the top rim particularly) of the frame designed to hold them.

107

In both (a) and (b) above when dealing with high-power positive or negative lenses, it must be stated once again that there is no alternative for judgement, practice and experience on the part of the optician. In any case, obviously the major considerations will be the technical ones associated with the performance of the lenses, and which lenses will give the best results for any particular case. So the frames and their role in the overall dispensing pattern tend to be less important relatively than the lenses.

7.6. Bifocal and Multifocal Dispensing

Once again, we are concerned solely with the question of the most suitable type and style of frame in which bifocals and multifocals can be dispensed. The major consideration is the fact that we have two or more areas of different focal powers mounted in the same frame. For different purposes the two eyes must be able to use each area binocularly as required. This requires that each area should be large enough to enable this essential requirement to be fulfilled.

¶3.8, ¶3.9 and ¶6.3 have already dealt with certain aspects of this matter. The dispenser should always bear in mind one fundamental consideration. A lens shape **must** be supplied with sufficient size and depth to enable the two or more areas to be placed in the frame so that the patient can see adequately with each. Particularly this applies to the depth of the lens. Total size or width is not so important, as the eyes are more concerned with vertical rather than horizontal movement.

A supra frame has an optical advantage for there is less obstruction to the field of vision in the lower part of the lens. The eyes can therefore use a lower portion of lens nearer the periphery, in a lens which is unobstructed by a rim. This enables a slightly shallower lens shape to be used in a supra than in a rimmed frame.

7.7. Peripheral Vision through Lenses

The standard procedure in sight-testing is to determine the lens or lenses which give the sharpest macular visual acuity in each eye for the purpose required (usually distance at 6 metres or 20 feet, and near at 33 cm.). Some slight adjustments for the sake of binocular comfort may have to be made to the monocular findings.

The whole area of the lenses is in use however when the spectacles have been dispensed, and even that portion of the extra-spectacle field around the outside of the frames is in use. Certainly, sharp visual acuity in the macular area is vital, but this is only part of the whole. The peripheral regions of the field are at times almost as important, particularly for driving, or for any occasion when detection of movement out of the direct line of fixation is needed. It is appreciated that binocular vision is normally achieved with the two eyes, but a car overtaking another car in the outside lane, for instance, will cause a response in the peripheral field of one eye only of the driver of the first car.

A spectacle frame will inevitably provide a certain amount of scotomata (blind spots or areas) which can prove very difficult and even dangerous in this context. In particular the scotomata due to the thick sides of library frames are very troublesome. Motoring organisations have on many occasions made representations to various optical bodies with a view to discussing means of dealing with the problem, but to no avail. This is one of the main pressures as to why larger and larger eye sizes are requested and, as will be appreciated, is purely a dispensing matter, the refraction having little bearing upon it.

7.8. Spectacles in Use

It might be a useful exercise to look at the matter from the point of view of the patient, and to try and determine what purpose spectacles are to serve. Firstly and obviously, they must be capable of providing adequate vision. The point is made in ¶7.7 that at times the peripheral vision is almost as important as the foveal vision.

The second requirement by the patient will probably be the comfort of the spectacles in wear. He must not be conscious of the weight of the frames in use, or at least not to the point of being so aware of the weight that it causes discomfort. A certain amount of awareness of the frame will be inevitable, more so at times than at others. With ladies who only wear spectacles for occasional use (e.g. presbyopic cases), the "marking" of the nose by the pressure of the spectacles resting thereon is a cause of considerable distress, and much complaint is levelled at the glasses on this account. Partly this is a combination of a suitable frame style and of the correct fitting, but again is exacerbated by too large a lens size. However, undoubtedly the main cause of this trouble is incorrect fitting of the frame.

The next point might well be the after-care of the spectacles. Most patients need to be told to return to the optician if there is any trouble of any sort, either relating to the lenses or to the frame. It is often not possible to determine whether either will be satisfactory until some days have elapsed and the person concerned has been able to try them. Most patients need to be told to return after a period of time for a check on the fitting and comfort, particularly with plastics frames which usually warp in use. The patient should also receive some sort of instruction on the care of the spectacles—to put them on and to take them off for instance with both hands—so as to avoid damage to one joint or to one side. Simple instructions of this sort on the use of the spectacles can prevent much abuse of the frames and can improve optician-patient relationship very considerably. Some opticians issue small booklets on these lines, or make a practice of sending postcards to patients advising them of the benefit of calling for a periodical check-up on their spectacles.

7.9. Confidence of the Patient

Reference has been made before on several occasions to the fact that the supply of spectacles (both frames and lenses) is an artistic as well as a technical matter. Equally it has been stressed that the patient plays an active part in the choice, and even to a certain extent, in the fitting of the spectacles.

Of equal consideration is the confidence that the patient has in the optician. This may be acquired either by knowing the person over a period of time, by dealing with members of his family, by undertaking a repair, or some other service. More usually it is on the basis of the impression which is created in his mind by the attention he receives at the time of his visit to have his eyes examined and spectacles provided.

Almost invariably the first person he will encounter when entering the optician's premises is the receptionist. The importance of a cheerful, attentive attitude cannot therefore be over-emphasized. The appearance of the premises is equally important. A dingy, dull, untidy, unwelcoming effect is very detrimental to the establishment of good relations.

At the time of the supply of the spectacles, almost invariably as a result of a sight-test, an interview is undertaken between patient and optician. It is essential to instil a sense of confidence and harmony between the two. The difficulties that flow from a lack of such confidence or from doubts that may arise are most unfortunate.

It must be remembered that we are dealing with the most important of man's five senses—his sight. Most people are very apprehensive of anything connected with their eyes, and will often go to extreme lengths to avoid having to seek advice or attention in case the advice they receive is unwelcome.

In years past there was a most definite psychological objection to the wearing of spectacles, as this was considered "ageing". Most people approaching middle age do not like having to wear spectacles, and resent the implication of age which presbyopic corrections automatically imply. Other age groups also have similar objections. Whilst not so prevalent nowadays, probably due in no small measure to the advent of smarter and more fashionable frames, this attitude of mind still exists.

As opticians we therefore have three functions to perform, assuming that the prescription is correct.

The first function is to reassure the patient particularly if elderly that his sight is not deteriorating, and that any fears in this direction are unfounded

The second function is to overcome the natural antagonism to the use of glasses which the implication of advancing years implies. There are many ways in which this can be done. The more diplomatic and helpful the optician is in carrying this out, the better will he be in doing his work.

The third function is to help the patient choose a pair of spectacle

110

frame which he (or she) will like. This may be phrased in a number of ways—which will suit him, which will enhance his physical attributes, which are smart and modern, or any one of the great number of imponderables which go towards flattering the individual's conception of what he is and what he looks like.

This is the most difficult of the optician's functions, and yet probably the most important. In fact, many opticians hand over this part of their work to younger colleagues if possible, especially when dealing with younger patients. At times, the delegating of such responsibility is not possible, so the receptionist is brought in to give advice and to offer encouragement either to patient or to optician.

The important point however is that if confidence is not instilled in the person, he will either not wear his spectacles; or he will wear them with reluctance and will grumble about and decry them to friends and relatives; or he will return them to the optician and complain of discomfort, unsuitability, or some other real or fancied difficulty.

This paragraph 7.9 on the necessity of gaining the confidence of the patient has been left till last. However, it is so important that it might well justify a chapter to itself.